"The best psychotherapy is deeply interpersonal and intersubjective for both patients and their therapists. Their relationships become saturated with reciprocal and complementary feelings and thoughts, especially their hopes and disappointments. As a devoted maverick, Dr. Stewart Aledort shares his clinical experience with patients who are 'difficult' and 'hard to reach.' He uses his own flawed self in the service of helping others heal their wounds of neglect and indifference. This exceedingly honest report is liberating, empowering and constructively provocative."

Earl Hopper, *PhD, Series Editor*

"With the tenacity of a bulldog and the warmth of a loving and available mother, Dr. Stewart Aledort, in his new book, treats his readers to a fresh, stimulating, and provocative account of his unique work with early-life emotional deprivation, trauma, and disappointment. He has the unique gift of working with misplaced loyalty, archaic grandiosity, somatic feelings, hidden excitement, and the deep and inconsolable parts of his patients. He does so with courage, boldness, creativity, respect, honesty, and, most of all, acceptance and kindness. Stewart provides his readers with an abundance of clinical examples and wisdom culled from his 50 plus years of clinical experience. Readers will return to their groups with renewed curiosity, understanding, and courage."

Jerome S. Gans, *MD, Distinguished Life Fellow, American Group Psychotherapy Association and American Psychiatric Association*

"In this very interesting book, Stewart Aledort details his unique understanding of how group therapy is best practiced. Deeply influenced by the work of Melanie Klein and Margaret Mahler, Dr. Aledort begins with the premise that for therapy to proceed, the patients must meet and accept the deeply, preverbal unconscious parts of themselves. Using interviews, case examples, and theoretical presentations, Aledort lets us see why he does what he does. At the end, we are given a touching view of the man as he approaches retirement."

J. Scott Rutan, *PhD, Past President, AGPA; Retired, Harvard Medical School; Massachusetts General Hospital Department of Psychiatry*

"This book is the story of a theory and the man behind that theory who single-handedly developed controversial ideas and practiced them. In an admirable and vulnerable way, Aledort candidly admits his belief the therapist is the most important person in the group, the group cannot be trusted initially, and the preverbal wish for fireworks animates every group patient. Blended with his personal story, including a backstage look at his retirement following the death of his wife, he explores

themes of sexuality, shame, narcissism, and aggression through use of rich case examples. These are absolutely new ideas offered in an absorbing way."

Joseph Shay, *PhD, CGP, AGPA-LF, Lecturer on Psychiatry, Department of Psychiatry, Part-time, Harvard Medical School; Editorial Board,* International Journal of Group Psychotherapy

"The author of this book is practically a legend to many members of the American Group Psychotherapy Association. During the last thirty years, Dr. Stewart Aledort's annual training presentations, along with his live group therapy demonstrations, have always been well received and enthusiastically attended by admiring colleagues and students from all over the world, eager to learn more about Stewart's instinctive and innovative approach to group psychotherapy. An introduction to Dr. Aledort's uniquely creative style, along with his brash, extemporaneous attitude toward group dynamics, usually results in group members discovering unique theoretical perspectives and innovative explanations, like the Omnipotent Child and the Passionate Bad Fit. Buy this book, read it thoroughly, and prepare yourself for an exciting journey through Stewart's unique theoretical model of group treatment. Chances are you will be surprised when you discover yourself eagerly ending up metaphorically on the container of Stewart's lap."

Philip J. Flores, *PhD, ABPP, AGPA-F, CGP; author*, Addiction as an Attachment Disorder *and* Group Psychotherapy with Addiction Populations

Advances in Group Psychotherapy

Advances in Group Psychotherapy presents an exploration of the work of Stewart Aledort in group psychotherapy.

The book covers key areas of Aledort's work in group psychotherapy, including theory and working with shame, anger, and aggression in the group. It includes theoretical and clinical cases from Aledort's work throughout, as well as new interviews which explore his most well-known theories. The book also explores Aledort's retirement from practice, with interviews exploring how he ended his group work after more than five decades.

Advances in Group Psychotherapy will be of great interest to all group psychotherapy and group analysis practitioners in practice and in training.

Stewart L. Aledort is a psychiatrist and group analyst based in Washington DC. He is a faculty member of the American Group Psychotherapy Association (AGPA).

Lee Kassan is a psychoanalyst based in New York City. He is a Life Fellow of the American Group Psychotherapy Association (AGPA).

The New International Library of Group Analysis (NILGA)
Series Editor: Earl Hopper

Drawing on the seminal ideas of British, European and American group analysts, psychoanalysts, social psychologists and social scientists, the books in this series focus on the study of small and large groups, organisations and other social systems, and on the study of the transpersonal and transgenerational sociality of human nature. NILGA books will be required reading for the members of professional organisations in the field of group analysis, psychoanalysis, and related social sciences. They will be indispensable for the "formation" of students of psychotherapy, whether they are mainly interested in clinical work with patients or in consultancy to teams and organisational clients within the private and public sectors.

Recent titles in the series include:

The Tripartite Matrix in the Developing Theory and Expanding Practice of Group Analysis
The Social Unconscious in Persons, Groups and Societies: Volume 4
Edited by Earl Hopper

Intersectionality and Group Analysis
Explorations of Power, Privilege and Position in Group Therapy
Edited by Suryia Nayak and Alasdair Forrest

Group Analysis
A Modern Synthesis
Sigmund Karterud

Tolerance - A Concept in Crisis
Psychoanalytic, Group Analytic, and Socio-Cultural Perspectives
Edited by Avi Berman and Gila Ofer

Advances in Group Psychotherapy
Living in the Passionate Bad Fit
Stewart L. Aledort
Edited by Lee Kassan

Advances in Group Psychotherapy

Living in the Passionate Bad Fit

Stewart L. Aledort

Edited by Lee Kassan

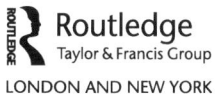
Routledge
Taylor & Francis Group

LONDON AND NEW YORK

Designed cover image: © Kara Aledort, Bears Den, Appalachian Trail, 2023

First published 2025
by Routledge
4 Park Square, Milton Park, Abingdon, Oxon OX14 4RN

and by Routledge
605 Third Avenue, New York, NY 10158

Routledge is an imprint of the Taylor & Francis Group, an informa business

British Library Cataloguing-in-Publication Data
A catalogue record for this book is available from the British Library

ISBN: 9781032705873 (hbk)
ISBN: 9781032705798 (pbk)
ISBN: 9781032705835 (ebk)

DOI: 10.4324/9781032705835

Typeset in Times New Roman
by codeMantra

Contents

Note from the Editor

I agreed to edit this book for Stewart Aledort for several reasons. I had been aware of Stewart and his way of working for many years. I had seen him lead workshops at the American Group Psychotherapy Association (AGPA) and at the Eastern Group Psychotherapy Society (EGPS) annual conferences. When I was editor of the EGPS journal *GROUP*, we published a long article (reprinted here) about his ideas, and I worked with him getting it ready for publication.

For reasons he talks about here, he had published very little material over his many years of practice. I think it would be a terrible shame if his unique ways of thinking and working were to get lost because they had never been written down. When we started working on the book, Stewart was close to retiring, and he has now shut down his group practice and his training groups and sees only a few individuals.

This is the last opportunity for students and new professionals (and seasoned professionals, too) to learn about this way of thinking about group and group treatment. I am proud to have been part of the process of collecting and presenting the work of Stewart Aledort.

Lee Kassan
Editor

Acknowledgments

This book could not have been written without the strength, vision, and fortitude of my late wife, Sheila. We both worked with patients, and she would join me at the annual AGPA events, to be with me at my Institutes and other panels and lectures. Looking to find her in the audience gave me the courage and chutzpah to believe I had great things to teach and share with my fellow therapists. We started to write the book that would inform therapists of the work I have been doing and at the same time enable me to take myself more seriously.

She hated to be in a group but managed to join one at every AGPA meeting we attended. People would kid us about how inseparable we were. They were right, yet there were times around her editing that the gloves would come off, and we both learned how to take a good punch, without hating or holding a grudge. I was so fortunate to be in such a loving, profound marriage with Sheila. As our work progressed, with the usual ups and downs, our relationship got closer, and at times I felt that we were one. But her keen editing, and her rejection of some of the words I used to examine my techniques and theories, reminded both of us that we were separate individuals trying to do a tough job. She continually made me take myself seriously, which I both admired and hated. This book is dedicated to her aliveness and her rather sudden and quick death three years ago, which forced me to reach out and find a new and wonderful editor, Lee Kassan, four years after her passing.

I was able to finish the book with the powerful and understanding help of my editor. His suggestion that he interview me for the first and last chapters worked well. It was painful to write and not have Sheila edit it but, as with most things, we do have the capacity to stay alive, to keep going, and to reinvent ourselves. As I do in my book, I had to take big risks, find a new identity, take myself seriously throughout, and grieve the loss of my life, my love, and my identity that was so wrapped up in hers. Grieving and separating are distinct experiences I had to negotiate to risk taking a new life force and a new, healthier identity. I had to tolerate my aloneness, which used to defeat me time and time again.

After a difficult emotional and physical two years of loss, I began to imagine how my own narcissism, which got funneled into my groups and my work, would be helpful in meeting new residents and learning to learn again, teach at times, and make new friends.

I want to thank Ms. Hillary Rubin, for finding me at Ingleside over a delicious book called *Horse*, by Geraldine Brooks. We met through the horse, and we both continue to laugh at our good fortune, I am not alone, and she has been of incalculable help in encouraging me and reading the developing manuscript. I listen carefully to her responses to delicate questions about the book. Hillary and I bring a great deal of joy, humor, and mutual respect for each other's courageous will to live a full life. We are living in a Passionate Good Fit.

My dearest and oldest friend, Dr. Martin Greenberg, was always the present, informative, reliable friend to help me out of some of my morasses and problems. He helped get me through Sheila's death, and I hope and know now that I was present for him through the recent death of his beloved wife, Janelle. There is a lot of death—that is what happens at our age, 85 and up.

Thanks go to Dr. Leslie Cohen and to Peter and Naomi Rosenblatt for their wonderful frequent brunches, Shep and Kate Shankman, Timothy Lindon, Wendy Velona, my wonderful grandson David Velona, and of course my daughter, Kara, who moved here from South Carolina to teach at the Lab School in DC. She has been the best support for me to be big, full of myself, and loving. Kara, with her optimism, her new job, and her love of life and for her father, was in a constant state of smiles and contentment about our relationship and our separate new identities. Among my old friends before Sheila's death, I want to thank the Rosenblatts, Randy Speck, Samantha Nolan, and my sister, Resa, and her husband, Arnie.

I want to thank my training group members, with me for over 30 years in New York and DC, for putting up with me and enjoying all our mutual growth and risk taking. Thanks to the AGPA faculty, such as Elliot Zeisel, Phil Flores, Joseph Shay, Scott Rutan, Yvonne Agazarian, and Ann Alonso, for their willingness to keep talking to me about theory and technique. They were unafraid to contradict me, to point out my harshness and my need to be more nurturing. All in all, I had great support, nurturing, love, and tough love from so many people.

In my present place of abode, Ingleside Retirement Home, I loved the questions and interest in my book from Steve and Monica Sindig, Rabbi George Dreissen, and Hillary's girlfriends Harriet Swankin, Judy Silber, and Judith Viorst.

Last but not least, big thanks go out to all my patients, who allowed me the honor of delving into their lives and trying to change some basic character traits. Most of them stayed until their happy graduation. They saved me when Sheila died. They allowed my narcissism to be used as a teaching tool, they borrowed some of my healthy narcissism, and they made the groups work and love and profoundly respect and take each other seriously. I will always love them, and they help me have healthy sleep at night, knowing I have been an important part of their lives. I sincerely thank you all for letting me be a part of your lives and time. We all toughened and loosened at the same time.

Respectfully and seriously, thank you all.

Stewart L. Aledort

Part 1

Theory

This section explores the concepts of the Omnipotent Child and the Passionate Bad Fit, and the stages of development that the group members, the therapist, and the group itself go through. The Omnipotent Child Syndrome is the first concept I wrote about to explain the essence of my group work. The early symbiotic mother dyad is shown with all its attendant frustrations, resistance, and relief. This section begins with an interview of me by the editor to explain my theories and techniques.

DOI: 10.4324/9781032705835-1

Chapter 1

Introduction to the Concepts of the Omnipotent Child and the Passionate Bad Fit

A conversation between Stewart Aledort and Lee Kassan

Discussion between Stewart and Lee explores and explains the basic concepts that are central to Stewart's way of working.

LK: I want to start with two definitions: the Omnipotent Child and the Passionate Bad Fits.

SA: In my way of thinking, the Omnipotent Child is the reservoir of all the early misattunements or Passionate Bad Fits in the mother–child dyad that reside in the body of the infant. The Omnipotent Child has all of the misattunements that reside in the right cerebral hemisphere of the brain.

LK: What makes it omnipotent?

SA: It's relatively indestructible; it demands a loyalty to it that in my mind is heroic, in that it's very, very difficult for someone to be disloyal to it, to the earliest experiences of the Omnipotent Child.

LK: It's omnipotent because it's in charge.

SA: And it's bigger than they are. It feels as if it's beyond their understanding.

LK: And it makes the decisions.

SA: It makes the decisions, and it puts enormous demands on you and is unrelenting. And in it is the early Kohut (1978) narcissism, and, as the bad fits get laid down in the right hemisphere, they have a somatic intensity that translates into a narcissistic power. That's part of what makes them so powerful. There's a narcissistic investment that becomes part of it. It becomes "This is who I am."

LK: It becomes part of the identity.

SA: Yes, a major part of the identity. It helps to define the person. As Cohen (2000) wrote, the most important thing for kids to do is to go back to an identity that they know, that stabilizes them. And one of the ways that you stabilize yourself as an adult is to keep living in the bad fit.

LK: And how do you define the Passionate Bad Fit?

SA: The term "Passionate Bad Fit" came out of the work with my group. They changed the language. I used to call it the Omnipotent Child, and then my patients would say, "You mean the Passionate Bad Fit."

DOI: 10.4324/9781032705835-2

The somatic passion that lays down the bad fit, and becomes part of who you are, and becomes the narcissistic piece of you, and the power it holds I call the Passionate Bad Fit because it is passionate, is a fit between mother and child and their bodies, and it is all-powerful. It's a reflection of the Omnipotent Child. It's the way it's portrayed to the therapist and the patient.

LK: Let me see if I have this right: The early bad fit with the mother is passionate because it contains a level of excitement and energy that is almost irresistible.

SA: And it comes from the body.

LK: It resides in the body. The new good fits are never going to have the level of energy and excitement that the old bad fits have.

SA: That's right. The new relationship will have safety and trust and maturity, but it will not have the drama of the old bad fit. It's the drama that stirs up the narcissism, that stirs up the soma, the body, that keeps alive the Passionate Bad Fit. It's the most magnificent thing that's ever happened to them, that they keep needing to repeat.

LK: That reminds me of how often patients will say, "I met this new guy, but he's so boring."

SA: That's a classic! And they choose someone in the group who can't stand them! "That's the one I want!" It's always that way. And I try to help them understand why it's always that way. I think a lot of therapists don't go as deeply as I do. They only go to the level of trying to help them understand.

LK: I don't think that patients have a comprehensive explanation of why the new adult relationship feels so boring.

SA: And it is! It is boring, compared to the fireworks. And we're always looking for fireworks.

LK: Okay, so now let's go into how you work, and the rationales for it.

SA: The biggest rationale behind the way I work is: after reading Margaret Mahler (1968), it became very clear to me that what was missing in a lot of groups that I participated in, or watched develop, was any attention paid to the preverbal period. It might be noted by the therapist, but it was never pursued or gone into. I said to myself, "What happens if I set up a group that would deal with the earliest preverbal period? How do I do that? How do I set that up?"

If you don't deal with that earliest period of your life, then all your behavior will still be controlled by the Omnipotent Child. And you'll always be running behind; he'll always be ahead of you, because he won't let it go by himself. The only way to let it go is for the patient to understand where it came from, and why they're holding on to it.

I realized this after many years of running groups by myself, and seeing that, no matter how well people did, they still held on to a piece of negative behavior that bothered them. Even if they had changed their job, or gotten a better marriage, they still held on to it. And a lot of people I saw had previous treatment—three, four, five, six years of treatment—and none of them got to the core. They got some changes on the outside but never got to the core.

And I felt after reading Margaret Mahler (1968) and Melanie Klein (1946) and watching Elvin Semrad in Boston do his thing about "Come into my lap" that I must get the groups to reexperience all the emotions of that wordless experience through the creation of the fantasized "lap" between the therapist as the mother of symbiosis. And the patient as a newborn baby.

LK: You got that from him.

SA: Absolutely. I got the okay to be in his lap. In fact, I presented a case to him of a young bi-polar lady, and she came in and the first thing she said was, "Santa Claus!" And she jumped into his lap, and started hugging him, and I figured, *That's it, I'm done. This is freaking me out.* It really was funny. He was great, and he said, "I'm not Santa Claus, but if you want me to be Santa Claus, what would you do with Santa Claus?" And I said to myself, *That's how it is! You don't run away from it, you build on it. They're telling you a story—build on it.*

LK: Move into it and not away from it.

SA: That's right, because this is the beginning, the tip of the iceberg. That's where I got the notion of the lap. When I saw him work with that woman, I said to myself, *My God, he knows how to get her to tell her story!* And an important part of the story is "I never had a lap. I need a lap."

LK: She literally sat in his lap.

SA: She didn't sit, she jumped!

LK: But you do it metaphorically.

SA: Yes, I do! Nobody jumps in my lap! One time, I was giving an institute in Boston, a demonstration, and there was a therapist in the audience who had seen me perform this six or seven times, and he said, "This time, Aledort, I am sitting in your lap! What are you going to do about it?" He gets up out of his chair, and he comes within two feet of me, a big, huge guy. We're talking, and I'm waiting for him to jump in my lap. He never did! I said, "You're welcome to jump in my lap, I can hold you," and he said, "I just needed to know that I was welcome," and then he walked away.

When I give a talk, there are many people in the audience who say, "How do I take a guy who's 200 pounds in my lap?" and I say, "You don't! It's in your mind, and in the patient's. He's not in your lap physically." I want to make that absolutely clear.

I was thinking, "How do I arrange this?" because I thought it was the most important thing. I decided in my mind that the new group that I run will become infants. I will see them as infants, and I become Mahler's mother of symbiosis.

Then for me, it was a challenge, because my notion of being the center, or crucial, was at first very unclear to me. Do you remember the movie *Taxi Driver*, with Robert DeNiro? He says, "You talkin' to me?" I said to myself, "That's the way to do it. Everybody is talking to me." And that felt good to me.

LK: What year was that?

SA: It was about 20 years ago. It was shortly after that I joined the AGPA. I wanted to have something of my own to talk about. I didn't want to be influenced by other people, and I stayed alone.

LK: That's curious, because you were obviously influenced by Semrad, and Mahler. What was your objection to being influenced by other people?

SA: I don't know. That's a good question.

LK: What occurs to me is that you were just formulating these ideas, and maybe they felt kind of fragile, and not ready to be exposed and potentially influenced by other people.

SA: Or criticized. So when I did start leading groups at AGPA using this model, over time people did help me move from a phallic DeNiro character, to a much more female mixture of Anne Alonso and Yvonne Agazarian and Margaret Mahler, people like that. I had to go through a metaphorical change internally, to go from the masculine, phallic leader, to a....

LK: To the nurturing mother.

SA: Right, to the inviting mother, with the inviting lap. I can't tell you when the lap came into existence, whether it was related to this shift, from phallic to feminine, but it had to be around that time, that I was able to *allow* a lap to come into my work, and to *be* a lap.

As a result of that, what I noticed was that there I had nine infants and me, in the group. At the beginning, I had some co-therapists, but I realized that I do better by myself. I remember having a long talk with Anne Alonso, who came as a consultant to the Washington School. I asked her about co-therapists and she said, "I never had a co-therapist. No one can keep up with me. When I run a group, I run the group." She said, "Stewart, I see exactly the same thing in you. You're fooling yourself by thinking you need a co-therapist. You don't need anyone." That gave me the confidence to do this on my own. I did have co-therapists from time to time. Some worked, some didn't work. Most of the time I did it by myself and that's worked out fine.

LK: How do you select people for the group?

SA: It's very simple. I have a whole evaluation process that I keep as simple as possible. I get a lot of referrals from people who want group therapy. I rule out people who are acutely suicidal or acutely psychotic—I don't take them in. I don't take anybody in the group who's litigious, who has a history of lawsuits. I have no interest in being sued, because my stuff is so controversial. "He wanted me in his lap! He wanted to fuck me! I'm suing him!"

So those are the criteria. The rest are people who have an ability to have some insight, who can take a look and see who they are. But that's not necessary. There are people I took who didn't have that ability but developed it over time. During the evaluation session, I look for any story they're telling me that has the Omnipotent Child or Passionate Bad Fit in it and see how they work with it.

The other thing is that I get them to try to talk about me. One of the things I see with patients who had many previous therapies is when I ask them, "How did you feel about your therapist? How did your therapist feel about you?" They say, "That never came up," and I'm amazed. I'm amazed at the number of people who went through therapy and got discharged as fine, and they never got into the transference. The therapist never stated that he/she was the most important person in the group and believed it (Aledort, 2002).

LK: I think that might have been before the relational shift that's happened in the analytic world…

SA: Yes, yes.

LK: …and if you asked them now you'd find that many more therapists actively address that material.

SA: Yes, but that was my experience. So part of my goal was getting them to talk about how they feel about me, and how they feel about my room. It's usually two sessions before they come into the group, and I ask if they've had any dreams about me, or any fantasies. I try to increase the relational experience, and at the same time I let them know that I'm going to be the most important person in the room.

LK: You're letting them know that the relationship between the two of you is going to be part of the work.

SA: That's correct. One of the things I do at the beginning, when the newborns are there, is I make it clear, when they start talking to each other, I stop them and I say, "You think you're here for Bobby, and Jane, and Carol. You're here for *me*. I'm the only person in your life who matters right now" That's how I start establishing that I am the mother of symbiosis and you're all my children, and I come first. These other kids, they don't matter.

People ask me, "How do you develop the group culture?" and I say, "The group culture is, what is it like to share this mother?" and that the other people don't mean anything now but will later on. That first experience can go for almost a year, in a once-a-week group. I do some individual work, with me as the center. "How do you think I would feed you, when you're hungry? How would you let me know that you're hungry?" If they look dazed, like "What are you talking about?" I would say,

> I'm asking you questions for which the answers are in your body, and we're trying to get your body to help you put them into words. So I'm going to ask you things that are related to your body, but they also have words attached that you didn't know existed until now, with me.

Someone once said to me, "I don't know how you'd feed me, but I was at a museum, and I saw a beautiful sculpture of a woman alone in a room." I said, "What did that mean to you?" He said, "I don't know what it meant to me." I said, "I guess what it most likely meant to you is you must have felt so alone with your mother, so isolated from your mother, who forgot to notice when you were hungry. Maybe that wasn't even important to you." This was someone who had trouble with their weight most of their life, gaining weight, losing weight. We kept working like that, and I would try to help them move from the inchoate, wordless, and somatic experience to words. I help them to find the words.

LK: And give them the language for their preverbal experience.

SA: Yes. And that seems to be very powerful. And that's how the group becomes a group. They're all waiting and knowing that at some point they'll be able to go from their preverbal to verbal, and they're all interested in how we get there. The guy before got there through a painting. Somebody got there through music. Somebody wrote a poem and got there. Somebody just cried. I had a patient who cried for three weeks, never stopped crying, and I asked him what he was crying about. He said, "I have no idea, but that's the way I was like." I said, "Well, your body was telling you how sad you were, or how sad your mother was, more likely." And then we found out later on that he was born after her beloved brother died. So she was in grief during his pregnancy and birth.

And so it comes together. And we keep working on that for at least a year. Every time someone tries to jump ahead, I pull them back. I say, "You're being precocious. You're not out of my arms yet. Why do you want to jump out of my arms? Come on back." We can appreciate the back-and-forth that goes on: the anger…

LK: Just as with a real child who wants to pull away and run off, and the mother literally pulls him back.

SA: That's right. Someone who shuts up, I say for them, "I'm not eating anymore because I don't like the way you feed me." And they say, "Goddamn you, that's right. I don't like the way you feed me. And I don't like all these other children. Why do you have to have all these fucking children?"

So we do that for about a year, and then somebody in the group defines the second phase of development by saying in his own way that he's ready. For example, I had flowers in my office, and this guy said, "The flowers are in my way, so I'm going to move them." I said, "No you're not. I like the flowers just where they are." He was pissed, just pissed. About a year later, he said, "Can I move the flowers?" I said, "I think you're ready to move the flowers." And that ushered in the phase of separation–individuation, because he had been more able to talk about the preverbal stuff. It went from, "I'm moving the flowers" to "Can I move the flowers?"

Separation–individuation goes on for a long time. That gets into the developmental phases.

LK: What are the rest of the phases?

SA: Well, separation and individuation is a big one. It starts off with a kind of "hatching," like the guy who wanted to move the flowers. I describe it to them this way: "You're not in my lap just to be fed, you're in my lap to look around and see what's out there. You're on my shoulder, and you're looking out and noticing people." Some people at that point regress, and they become silent, and I'll say, "I think we jumped ahead too soon. I think you still need to be in my lap, to be fed, to be held. I don't think you're ready yet to take a look outside."

Precocious behavior comes in all different forms. There was a guy I wrote about who tried to see me. He was a friend of someone I had treated. Every time he called, he said, "My friend said I should come to your group. How much is it?" I told him and he said, "It's too much!" and he hung up. This went on for years, and he kept hanging up. He finally came into the group. When he was in the lap, he was thrilled by it, but he had to get out. It was too confining. It was too intimate, and he didn't like it. He wouldn't use that word, but he would say, "I feel trapped, I feel claustrophobic. I feel like your arms are too big. I feel like your lap is too deep. I can't get out of it. Maybe I could jump out of it." I said, "Yes, I think you've been living most of your life trying to jump out of places, and never settling into places." And suddenly, he would jump out of my lap, not physically, and start dealing with the women in the group, and he would get killed by the women. The women would say, "You're rude, you're crude, you're disgusting, you're too sexual." I kept saying, "You need to come on back."

Through that kind of thing, I began to appreciate that rapprochement is so important. The lap has to be there all the time, for as long as the group survives, because one needs it at various times. So what I would do is I would call him back, and say,

> Let me help you deal with the women. But first, get on my shoulder, and tell me which women you see, and which ones you like and which ones don't you like. And if you like Mary, tell me what you want to say to Mary.

Meanwhile, Mary is in the room, listening. She might say, "What am I, chopped liver?" And I would say,

> I'm trying to teach him how to have a discussion with you, so you don't have to throw him back in my lap, because your problem is that you throw everybody back. You need to appreciate, if you come into my lap, why you can't put up with someone who isn't just perfect.

Through the interaction, as with everybody else, I work with it. I go back and forth between the Omnipotent Child and the Passionate Bad Fit.

The phrase "Passionate Bad Fit" came from my patients. They changed it from the Omnipotent Child. I remember a group in particular who said, "The Omnipotent Child sticks in my throat. I prefer the 'bad fit'." And then someone said, "You mean the 'Passionate Bad Fit'." It sort of evolved over time.

LK: This guy you were just talking about, I would say that this is a guy with an avoidant attachment style.

SA: You're totally right.

LK: Do you find attachment theory of any use to you?

SA: Yes, I do, and I use it. I don't use it as a major way of thinking, but I certainly try to understand what the attachments were. And that takes place in the lap, and from then on. Attachment theory is very important (see Cohen & Rogovin, 2000).

LK: You talk a lot about the room.

SA: Yes. The room is very important, which I think a lot of therapists don't appreciate. I had a lovely office in Georgetown, but it was on the street, and there was always noise—cars, cops, fire engines. At the beginning, when they're infants, what I noticed was sometimes they would leave the door open from the waiting room to the group room, and I decided to see how long that would be, and so I didn't get up and close it. What's interesting is they kept it open, but they never talked about how disturbing the sounds were in the office. They made it clear to me later on, as the group got older and more mature, and they were able to go back and talk about it, that leaving the door open and not noticing the noise was the essence of the autistic phase of Mahler's theory, which is "We are one. We are *not* separate. We are just one. So the rest of the world doesn't exist."

LK: So there was no boundary.

SA: There was no boundary. It was beautifully shown in the office. Then, as we moved on to separation–individuation, and we created a boundary, then the door was always closed. Then they started noticing the room, and they started saying, "It's too hot in here," or "It's too cold in here," or "The light hurts my eyes," or "There's too much goddamn noise in here. Why do you have the office in Georgetown? Are you some wealthy son of a bitch?" And it became very clear to me that the room then became the mother–infant dyad. It became that early experience of the mis-fit between the mother and the child, and their bodies together, and the feeding experiences, and the nursing experiences, and changing the diaper experiences. I began to interpret the dyad in that response. For example, a woman would say, "I just don't like that," and I would say,

> You've never liked *anything* that you had to be part of. You'd always complain about a dress you bought that never fit correctly. How can you buy a dress that doesn't fit? What made you buy it? And you're always complaining about your shoes aching. How come you don't get new shoes?

LK: So in addition to the relationship to you that recreates a lot of the early stuff, the office itself is another vehicle for that.

SA: For interpretation and re-creation. A new member would come into the group, a very tall guy, and he'd say, "You know, these lights are too harsh.

So, Stewart, could you change the lights?" The group said, "Forget it, buster. You're in the room forever. Forget the lights. You might as well begin to understand that it's you and your mother and your body. So sit down and be part of the group." And he was shocked, but it was very helpful to him.

LK: So when you start a group, do those people all stay in the group together throughout the life of the group? Do you bring in new people or not?

SA: Yes. That's a very important thing. The group is open-ended, but my experience is that a group within the group forms, a solid core of people, usually about 5, and they become the stabilizing force that moves through all the developmental phases together. Then there's an outer ring of 2 or 3 people who come and go. Some leave prematurely, and a new member comes in, and sometimes they get into the core group and sometimes they don't. But the group then becomes the symbiotic mother. The small group within the group takes on my job, and becomes the mother of symbiosis, and a new member coming in has to deal with them.

They want to treat the new member the same way I treated them. They need to look at the earliest experiences, and as they do that they become more and more confident, they begin to notice some interim changes, and they begin to notice they're living more in a Passionate Good Fit.

Then that gets us to the most important phase, which is, how do you move? How do you ultimately get from a Passionate Bad Fit to a Passionate Good Fit? How do you get both feet in there? And that takes years.

Right now I have a bunch of groups that are very close to that point. Some of that has to do with *my* ending, because I've been sick and been more open about it. We get into risk-taking—What is a risk? How do you take risks? How can you feel disloyal to the heroic early Omnipotent Child, and still feel good about yourself? How do you live without shame?

LK: You mentioned shame. How do you conceptualize shame?

SA: Shame is an internal failure, to not allow the person you love to keep loving you.

LK: Can you elaborate on that?

SA: Let's take an example. Almost every patient, when they're the newborn, and they put it into words, they almost always blame themselves for their mother's failures. "I didn't let her hold me well enough." "I screamed too much." "I fidgeted too much."

LK: "I was a difficult baby."

SA: And some people who I actually worked with had colic, and another had a rash so the mother couldn't hold the baby, and so they blame themselves. And throughout their history, they do the same things to their wives, and husbands, to their bosses. They're always putting the blame on themselves.

The other thing that they do, which is part of being a good child, a wonderful child, is take on the parents' shame, to allow the shame to be induced into them.

LK: To try to heal the parents, so they can get what they need from the parents.

SA: Right. But they end up with the shame, and the humiliation. They end up with the sense of failure. And I see it in every phase of development that we go through. We have to go through this shame/humiliation cycle, and then we see it in the group in different ways. Group members can shame each other, and they accept it rather than putting it back. I say, "You've got to put it back. You can't let her get away that. Put it back into that person." And she's saying "Wait. I don't want it. Why give it to me? I didn't give him anything." I say, "Yes, you did." And then she was able to talk about *her* humiliation, and he began to feel that he had started to put it back.

    So part of the healing process is putting back the shame and humiliation, that you own, back where it belongs. That gets replayed in the group, as well as in their lives.

LK: When do you start trusting the group, and what does that mean?

SA: I remember when Scott Rutan and I had a whole big discussion. He came to Washington to be a consultant, and it turns out I was *his* consultant, when he was running a group. The way he worked, I said,

> You trust the group, so you can sit back and not say much at all, at the beginning. You just let the group say whatever they want. I don't. I don't think the group has the ability, because they're newborns, to do what's necessary to keep the group functioning. You think they do, because you don't see them as newborns. You see them as adults. A 40-year-old man coming in with previous history and therapy, you assume he's mature enough to run the group. I don't, and that's where we differ.

I don't trust the group until they're able to be in my lap and be able to navigate separation–individuation. And once you begin to navigate that, and when you have trouble to come back to the lap, then I can trust you. I think you are now capable of helping yourself and of helping others in the group.

    So at that point, I recede, give up a lot of the symbiosis, and the core group develops that takes on the symbiosis, without shame or humiliation, and at that point, I become more of a transference object. At that point, I could become the father, the mother, or whatever.

LK: The sibling.

SA: That's right. The sibling, the boss, the wife, whatever. I become a transference object, which I stay for a while, but I always have the lap. One of the things I've noticed recently is that when I first conceived of the lap, I conceived of it as for a needy infant. Now I see it as for an overworked, stretched, highly anxious, well-producing adult, who needs a break. He can't do it, he can't keep doing it. So there are many people to whom I'd say, "It's okay for you to come into my lap and admit that you're stressed out, that you need a lap. You need to stop for a minute. You're working too hard. You're taking too much responsibility."

So the lap then, for some people, becomes a place to keep going back to, to be taken care of as they take more risks in their life.

LK: Like the oasis in the desert.

SA: Well put. That's right. It serves many purposes, many functions.

LK: What are the challenges for you, in working this way?

SA: In the beginning, I couldn't sustain DeNiro. It got out of hand. As I gave institutes at AGPA, which were filled with very sophisticated people, they said, "You can't do it. You're getting too angry."

LK: Too much aggression.

SA: Too much aggression in DeNiro's taxi driver. So I began to try to be less aggressive, and the biggest change for me was to go from phallic to feminine. I managed that by marrying my wife, Sheila, and she was able to say to me,

> You know, in a way you're not taking yourself seriously as the thinker. You're not the clown. You should take yourself seriously. You say yes to everybody and everything. You have things to say; you have things to write. Say them.

There was something about that that allowed me to be a different kind of person, because Sheila was able to work with me about it.

LK: She gave you a model of what kind of mother to be.

SA: I think so. I don't think I had one. My previous relationships did not have one. She allowed me to be a woman who was respected, who enjoyed being a woman. She helped me move from DeNiro to the mother. So it opened up a whole new ballgame for me—what's it like to really understand women? Before that, I don't think I spent enough time trying to understand women, and who they are, and what they need.

LK: So you made that transition, and what are the challenges now?

SA: How long do I keep working, is the biggest one—retirement.

LK: How old are you now?

SA: I'm going to be 85. But I never felt like it before—I always felt young, until I got sick. And then when my wife died, it was a very difficult period. So I moved into a residential community, assisted living, and at first I hated every minute of it. Slowly but surely it's become okay now. I had to deal with that while running my groups, grieving without a hug during the COVID pandemic, without being able to honor my wife with a funeral service, and then some health issues. I would scream to myself, "I need a hug —where are you?"

LK: These are challenges in your life as a whole. I want to focus more on the challenges of the work itself.

SA: The biggest challenge is that my patients are all getting better and moving on, and I'm ending my life. Dealing with that. And wondering if I can be disloyal to my work—how do I stop this work?

The biggest difference is this—I started sharing things about myself with the group, which I never did before. That started with Sheila's death. I couldn't share it.

LK: The group is seeing things in you, and you have to explain them.

SA: Yes, I did, and in more detail than I ever imagined I would. That surprised me, because I've always been against therapists exposing themselves. I always thought that they lost some of their therapeutic zeal and expertise when they do that. But here I am talking about the death of my wife. It was during the pandemic so they knew I was living somewhere else. I was circumspect about that, but I would answer many more questions than I ever did before.

LK: What effect do you think that had?

SA: I think it brought the group very close together. Most important, it allowed the group to take risks themselves, about what *they* reveal. There were a lot of secrets that came out.

LK: Wasn't that interesting, though?

SA: Yes, that it had such a profound effect. And a lot of hidden sexual fantasies.

LK: That's so interesting to me, that your disclosure led to that. There's a big controversy now about how much self-disclosure to do. In fact, a lot of people have reported over the last 18 months [of the pandemic] revealing more than they were used to, and sometimes more than they were comfortable doing, but doing it anyway. It's the first time that we are all in the same trauma as our patients.

SA: That's right. You're correct. After a while, I found it very relieving for me, where the group was sort of *my* lap, and I had to always be careful that I wasn't misusing it, or abusing it. I was always watching myself as I was talking about these things.

LK: Of course, because that's the guideline—is this for them or for you?

SA: I think the thing that's most striking is the risk-taking. And that opened up the door for us to discuss why people take risks, why they don't take risks, and what risks have people been taking with each other in this room.

I have three groups that I'm running now. And one group member said to me,

> I know what you're doing. I figured you out. You're preparing us, so that when you die, or retire, that we're on the road to a very full life. You're preparing us as best you can before you leave us. So what do you have for us?

I said, "I have three therapists that you're going to interview, to see if you want to work with any of them." They want to know what I can give them as I'm ready to leave, and what they can give me.

They're much closer, they're much more open and willing to talk about love, loving me, my loving them, the troubles they're having that interfere with the loving, and some of them say, "I'm going to get as much out of you as I can before you die." That's been a big change, the amount of self-disclosure, the risk-taking She's right—I am preparing them for the best life they can have, in very specific ways.

One woman, who's been looking for men, I ask her, "Why haven't you been looking for a man like me? Find someone like me." They're able to talk about loving me, what does it feel like, do I love them, how do I love them. It's warm and loving, but also tough. Somebody said, "How come we never talk about money in this group? We can talk about sex, but we never talk about money." So we end up talking about money.

Somebody says to me, "You use your narcissism all the time in here." And I say, "Yes, you're right." And she said, "How do I use my narcissism? Do I use it in a healthy way or an unhealthy way?" So we are now talking about risks, narcissism, and leaving. For instance, we ended up talking about a woman in the group who has sort of lived in the shadow, and she's been a very promiscuous lady, and nobody asks about it. I say, "How come nobody asks about her sex life? She tells me about it in individual sessions, but how come nobody wants to know about it?" I think people don't want to know about it because they want to stay small, narcissistically small, in their lives. They don't want to take those risks.

LK: My thought is that they don't want to be envied or envious.

SA: Yes, that's right, and that's come up. I work more in the narcissistic part of it by saying,

> Have you ever met anyone who can be so secretive, and deliciously small like this? She's a pro. Isn't she a pro? She's the most magnificent small, secretive woman we've had in this group for years, and she loves every minute of it.

I say to the others, "How are you the most magnificent in this room?" I'm going after what is their most magnificent piece, that they are hiding from other people how magnificent they feel about it, and where narcissism sits and attaches itself to these parts of themselves, as they're preparing to leave, as they're preparing for my ending of the group.

LK: You're reframing and redefining what narcissism can mean. I think for most people it's always a negative.

SA: I know that.

LK: So you're giving them an alternative definition, that this could be a positive thing.

SA: Absolutely. And we talk a lot about "healthy narcissism" versus "unhealthy narcissism." A lot of the time I'll bring it back to me. That's one of the things I also do—I become the object of desire. I think a lot of therapists, particularly women therapists, have a hard time being the object of desire. That's another piece in this. It's very important to work with this, the object of desire.

LK: Is there anything else we need to cover?

SA: I think it's really important to let people tell their stories, no matter what form it takes, and one of the roles of the therapist is to allow people to tell their stories. And how crucial it is for people, when they meet each other, or who are getting married, to tell their stories to each other. A lot of people don't tell their stories and then they're struck by surprise, guilt, anxiety, humiliation, shame. It's a way to cut down on the shame. I'm always thinking in group about how I can continue to get people to tell their stories.

LK: You try to do that early in their group participation?

SA: Early on. Right from the beginning. I say right at the beginning, "You're here to tell the story of your early feeding, your early experience. And then later on you'll tell your story many different ways." When patients have a lot of anxiety, I'll say, "Tell me what part of the story it fits with. Obviously you've had the anxiety before. Your body is holding it. What is the story around your anxiety? Please try to tell us the story."

I think that's important. Sometimes therapists forget to have people tell their stories. So at the end of my life, at the end of my role as a therapist, in my own way I'm telling *my* story. That's what we're doing here.

Chapter 2

The Stages of the Developmental Model

Stage I: Symbiosis and the Therapist's Lap

Each new member of the group is experienced as a newborn, which is explained to the member both in the consultation sessions and in the early group experience. I work individually with the new member and feel like the mother of symbiosis to the newborn baby. We try to interact with each other, and I let the members know that we are quite reliant on each other, as the other members have been with me. "I am the most important member of the group, and you are the most important new baby in the group." I comment on how they have presented themselves to me and the group. Like wearing a hoodie, slumped in the chair, sprawled out on the couch like he owns it, silent and trying to live in the dark. I work with their presentation and let them know that it is their way to let me know of the long overdue story of their earliest life, the one without words. They usually do not like those comments or being seen as a newborn baby in the group, but they do not leave. Why not? They are intrigued by my approach and my shameless grandiosity and never imagined that anyone, much less a group, would be interested in their wordless life. They are struck by how the body really tells the story instead of words. I let them know, "As we continue this work, you will be able to put words to that early period in your life."

As we try to talk to each other, the group takes in again their own early wordless life and identifies with the pain, sadness, and futility expressed by the new member. They then tell us about feelings in their body, such as blushing, talking loud, chest pain, boated feelings, constipation, eating disorders, and how their body was more an enemy than an ally. The new member yells,

> Go away, get out of my life. I want to leave this group. This is not for me. I don't like the way you look at me, or try to like me, or try to love me. You are full of shit.

The group says to the new member,

> Stop fighting him, and no, he will not go away, and he wants to help us get beyond seeing ourselves as damaged babies who cannot express ourselves in

DOI: 10.4324/9781032705835-3

words. This guy will help you do it. Like he is right now. You must have been pretty mad at your mother. You may have felt that she was disingenuous and did not feel real to you. You might have felt, like all of us, that we were not held the right way, that it was hard to feel loved and safe and relaxed. Our bodies kept telling us that, but we didn't know how to listen, much less what to do about it. We all felt helpless, scared, and unsafe. Otherwise, we would not be in this group with pain-in-the-ass Dr. Aledort.

As the sessions evolve, there is more one-on-one with me, as we try to identify the unsafe feelings and misattunements in this early wordless phase. There is very little actual memory before age 3 but, through our work, feelings of injury and tension begin to be explored. I slowly inject the idea of the therapist's lap as a safe place to learn and explore these somatic feelings and to feel safe this time. As expected, there is an enormous amount of hostility to this idea. The thought of having a lap feels preposterous to the new member, and so unsafe. Many memories get stirred up in this part of the work, all within the first year of the new member's entry into the group. Memories of failed intimacies with the mothering figure fill the room: how feeding was not predictable or easy; how cleaning of our bodies was not easy and relaxing; how being held hurt and felt claustrophobic at times. It was not clear who was the infant and who was the mother. Dealing with the mother's anxiety, her anger about being a mother, her depressions, and her attempts to love, all felt injurious to the new member. There was relief, the baby said later, that I was clear that I was the commanding figure in their life, even though there were other babies in the group. I made sure that I could incorporate all the feelings, good and bad, that the mother of symbiosis needed to do. She is symbiotic (Mahler, 1968) because they are merged, and I intensify that feeling by acting at times as if the other babies do not exist. All dialogue flows through me, not with each other, in the first year of the group. On occasion, there is slippage, and I cannot hold on to the symbiotic stance (the frame), and in fact defer to the other babies, while still trying to diminish the one-on-one talk among them. I tend to bring it back to me, with great annoyance and hurt feelings. "I came to this group for the others," they say. I say, "No, you came to this group for me and my reputation. And that's what you're getting. You'll soon be able to relate to each other, after we get through this wordless stage."

The role of the therapist during this phase is to be resolute, strong, and loving, and to learn how to listen to the babies, and try to experience with them a new merger that is not built on failures and shame. You, the therapist, must be willing to let the baby enter your body, to let the baby incorporate you as a different kind of mothering figure. You must try to figure out, with the help of the baby, the proper distance between you, and to pay special attention to signs of anxiety, injury, or hurt feelings in this intense one-on-one. The baby is usually willing to try out the concept of the lap when they feel more located inside of the therapist. You have to tolerate the baby's crawling inside of you and exploring your insides. If the therapist screws up, he must admit it was his fault and not the baby's. If the baby cannot be held, calmed, or soothed by the therapist, they must talk about how hard it is for both of them to feel satisfied with themselves and with each other. At this moment that is all they have. You can see early on, in some babies, the need to not satisfy the mother and to make her feel as frustrated as the baby is. Who supports the therapist during this intense year of the group with the new member? Sometimes it is the co-therapist; sometimes peer supervision, other colleagues, individual supervision; and sometimes your own rich fantasy life, as well as your own admiration of how wonderful and exciting and caring you are. I have always wanted to be a member in the group that I run.

Stage II: Separation and Individuation

When they are finally ensconced in the safe lap, the urge, both biological and psychological, for individuation comes alive. The babies start fidgeting, looking over your shoulder in their fantasy of being seated on your lap. They begin to notice the other, and the therapist must deal with his diminished role as the all-knowing symbiotic mother. They want to say hello to the others and assume that you will interfere and maybe even hurt them if they leave you. The other side is that they could feel rejected and unloved when you signal that enough is enough and you want them out of your lap. You may feel that they cramp your style now or would rather do something else for yourself. Can the therapist admit that it was time for him to do something different for his own needs, and it would be better right now if the baby tried to seek out and notice others? Can he admit to his narcissistic injury of not being the most important person in their life now? Can he admit to a narcissistic injury? He'd better get used to it, because there will be many more to come.

The therapist is now needed to hold both the baby's need to see the world and the need to stay safe. The therapist must be able to hold these two conflicting feelings at the same time and be able to digest and give back to the members the quandary he shares with them. This ability to expose to the babies your own internal dilemmas and soft spots allows the babies to continue the process of knowing the inside of the mothering figure as the babies tell the therapist and show the therapist their insides (Stolorow & Lachman, 1980). This is not the therapist exposing personal history in his or her life. This exposure comes from facilitating the ongoing work of mutual discovery that rarely happened in their life. Awareness of the other is profound, and some members have expressed their feelings with the sudden onset of tears that they cannot explain, sudden panic attacks, or an intense wish to leave the group, and the intense feeling of wanting to be held forever. The therapist holds and contains the strong reactions, by explaining that they suddenly notice a piece of themselves, a piece of identity that terrified them. They would have stayed merged with the symbiotic mother, at any cost, then feel and notice the burgeoning new identity, separate from the symbiotic mother.

This dynamic first plays out in many ways within the group. One group organized a special sub-group to climb a mountain, while leaving some others behind.

One of the rejected ones brought along a kerosene can and started a fire in their cabin. The rage was hot, the rejections intense, and the rejecting group was smug and unapologetic to the others. They did mourn their cabin, but not the others they rejected. This clear beginning of seeing their Passionate Bad Fit in stark daylight both amused them and terrified them.

One member, who turned out to be one of the most difficult to work with, struggled with me about moving some plants that were in the way of his seeing the rest of the group. I told him that the plants were mine, not his, and we were trying to figure out what belongs to each of us and how we negotiate that. This had always been his major narcissistic and grandiose conflict. "I can do what I want to do, and you have to accept it." He had very little empathy or acknowledgement of others and his impact on them. He could only bitterly complain of their impact on him. He did and then became aware of how he self-sabotaged his success, only to take refuge in his Passionate Bad Fit, with its toxic merger with his mother and father. There, in that refuge, which he sought out with me and members of the group, he was seen as being brilliant and carrying the family magnificence, while putting up with his Rumpelstiltskin childlike behavior.

He tried to run the group, and he and I had many conflicts about that. He was not going to usurp me, not on my watch. He could not tolerate the loss of grandiosity after he was pushed toward separation. He desperately needed to merge, to recapture his lost grandiosity. He got into huge fights with his mirrored female member of the group. She could outfox and outplay him. Both are my most painful failures in the groups. The theory did not work, the empathy and relatedness to the group did not work, and I did not make it work. I was too angry at these narcissistic, sadistic members. I was too caught up in my age-old fight with a highly narcissistic and successful older brother, who I can never get to treat me better, which brought out my sadism toward him. In retrospect, I was reliving my ongoing problems with my difficult brother, where we bring out the worst in each other.

It is so easy for the therapist to relive his issues with the group, and he needs a radar system to tell him when it is happening. Our need for supervision and continuous analysis is crucial in controlling this reliving. We then recapture our lost grandiosity, with shame as the springboard and organizer of it. That is the clue that is so easy not to notice. We are caught up in reclaiming the lost grandiosity that we do not notice the shame organizing recaptured grandiosity that we are basking in, usually at the group's and members' great cost. The phase of separation–individuation makes the therapist more vulnerable to this acting out, because it heralds the lost grandiosity and the need to recapture.

During this phase, there are many times when I have to ask a member to join me in my lap. Over time, the group will tell a member that he needs to get in the therapist's lap. We see this a lot with children with a precocious history, with members who are throwing around their shameful narcissism at the other members. The babies feel that they have been held back by the lap and have no interest in returning, even when asked. Yet their behavior demands that the therapist try to get the baby in the lap again. This struggle is intensified and leads to new material about their early life, and the babies having to contain their outrage, sadness, and despair in their early childhood. They are able to put words to this time. They begin to appreciate boundaries, to appreciate the power of the lap and their resistance to it, and the range of feelings that are inside of them. They can start talking and showing us how their bodies hold all these feelings.

> One member would move his arms like a rooster crowing, and was unaware of it until it was gently pointed out to him. He was able to say that he could never crow about anything growing up, that was left to his parents. He always felt that he underperformed, and never trusted his body to play competitive sports or to let him sleep at night. He did begin to crow, and the rooster disappeared from the group.

Stage III: Identity and Sexuality

This next phase, which is always lurking in the background noise of the group, heralds itself as members begin to notice the other members' sexual identity. For the first time, group dreams appear, with their feelings of titillation, curiosity, and excitement. Members are surprised by the excitement in the dreams, and how they rarely pay attention to their dreams. They then could begin to articulate how they either think about sex all the time or rarely think about it. The members try to decide whether the group is erotic or not. I ask them what they do with their new-found eroticism here in the group.

> One member, who earlier had spoken about how close and inappropriate his mother tended to be with him, jumped at the chance to be inappropriately sexual with the women in the group. He was like a ball of energy that ran the show, and he could not control that part of himself. The group, over time, demanded that he return to my lap and decompress all this pent-up sexual energy. He reluctantly came, and noticed a calming down of his anxiety and his eroticism. He found a safe harbor in the group. The coming and going from the lap gets understood as confusion about what it means to leave the lap and notice all this pent-up energy.
>
> They also notice that their brains are trying to understand and make sense of this phase. It reminds them of their own grandiosity and how it feels now that it resides in them, and they are free from the mothering lap. As they notice the changes in their minds and bodies, they wonder who they are. Members talk about a sense of isolation, curiosity, sadness, and fear of not knowing who they are now. I let them know that they are becoming aware of having lived in a Passionate Bad Fit for the last 5 to 8 years. They were as fearful of their freedom as of staying in the lap forever. They are incredulous when I allow and help them to leave the lap, but also remind them that the lap is here when they need it.
>
> (Aledort, 2003)

The difficulty of leaving the mothering figure distorts the separation process and corrupts the notion of the nurturing woman, or of the process of being held and loved. The group talked about how hard it had been for them to ask to be held and, most of all, how hard it was to love and be loved. They ended up with partners whom they could not love but could not leave. They tended to get rid of partners who could enable them and teach them to love. They did not know who they were without the Passionate Bad Fit. They selected partners in the group who would not give them what they wanted and therefore relived the anxious and defeated tension of their childhood. The unconscious motivation was to end up in the agony and safety of the Passionate Bad Fit. The partner is a vehicle to get and live there. It is the powerful and sad truth that most felt that their pain and injury was not being able to love their parents in a healthy way.

> One man expressed his love with a woman in the group, who had no real interest in exploring love with him or anyone else. She favored the slow, ongoing disappointment in her husband, and accepted it as a step better than her relationship with her mother. They had fantasies of meeting outside the group room, but it always ended in disappointment or hurt. It is only after almost two years of their relationship that they are able to learn more about themselves. Their relationship needed to happen for them as well as for the group. It opened the door to sexual longing and the need to love and be loved. They both can now just be sad.

Stage IV: Movement to a New Identity

Shame keeps the Passionate Bad Fit in place and shame keeps it alive. The Passionate Good Fit is kept alive by healthy narcissism, without shame as the organizer. Shame is a powerful organizer and can be eroticized and sought after. It is the ingredient that causes and keeps alive the somatic memory of the misattunements in human relationships. Shame is transported within families and projected onto family members. Those who accept the shame, the chosen ones, become, in fantasy, united with the lost grandiosity of infancy, which is coupled with implanted shame and aggression and eroticism that the chosen child carries to become his Passionate Bad Fit in later years (Morrison, 1989).

The search for lost grandiosity allows the continuation of the shame to lead to a very entangled, highly charged merger with a parent. The fantasized closeness with the parent, who is disappointed and hurt, temporarily soothes the narcissistic injury, and leads to temporary relief in the injury state. Both the parent and the child can feel more relaxed and healthily closer to each other in this period of rapprochement.

When further misattunements occur, and they invariably do, the regressive experience leads to the archaic grandiosity of Kohut (1978). This archaic grandiosity continues with more energy and more hurt and disappointment and ultimately ends up as the Passionate Bad Fit. The fantasy resolution of the continuous injuries, where shame takes over the process, leads to the formation of the Passionate Bad Fit neuronal structure located in the right cerebral hemisphere (Schore, 2002a).

How these formulations get played out in the dynamics of the group is the essence of both my technique and my theory. Clinically, we see people struggling to attach through the Passionate Bad Fit to others in the group. As they learn more about their early years, through working with me, and the shame intimately connected to the injuries, they experience relief that they can begin to put words to the wordless, somatically driven early years. They begin to try out my fantasy symbiotic-mother lap, I help them see through their individual reactions to me as the mother of symbiosis, how no one in the group ever had a safe, normal, healthy lap at their disposal. The lap sustains their need for a safe place and allows them the opportunity to scan the world and try to decide how they would like to begin some separation from the parenting figure.

Separation attempts are made in the group, and an enormous amount of information accompanies these experiences. As part of this process, they begin to figure out who they are and what their relationship is to others and to their bodies. As they struggle to put this task and conflict into words, I act as a narrative upstage voice for the group. I say,

> Imagine how hard it is for you to say that you need more space without feeling disloyal and terrified that the nurturing would cease and how you could be abandoned. You ask yourself, 'I cry, does she notice? I'm going to hold onto my bowel movements to feel bad about myself but still loyal to the merger. I will struggle with being fed, I will not allow her to hold me and give her pleasure. But I will always smile, play games with her, make her smile, and then feel a little crazy doing all this stuff that confuses me. I just want to go to sleep for a long time. The safety of my crib, the bottle that I drink from, and the thought that I am still merged, still loved, and still loyal all gently rock me to a delicious sleep. Can I do all these things?'

They struggle with the body as ally or enemy. They deal with disappointment and how little they know of themselves. They also note how little they know of their parents and family, and of the therapist.

This period of work usually leads to members working on their differences with each other, and the issues of gender and sexuality appear. This has led to many intense sessions, fights, romances, and intense yearnings. The stories of failed relationships, failed sexuality, and ultimately failed intimacy are present. The therapist reminds them all, repeatedly in many ways, that their experiences had a great deal to do with their living in the Passionate Bad Fit, which affects intimacy, identity, conflict resolution, and self-esteem.

Stage V: Crossing the River

In about the fourth or fifth year of our work together, a strong, firm nucleus of members, about four or five, become the healthy center of the group work. The therapist's role, which has been changing since the group started, now can take on new and different forms, that of consultant, transference object, and object of desire, but always with his lap available when members need one. When a member begins to cause havoc in the group, and feels anxious or lost and out of control, I beckon him back to the lap to quiet himself, and then to observe how others are reacting from the safety of my lap. Even the healthiest and busiest member sometimes needs the lap to rest and recover. The therapist allows and enables couples to form attachments, and members to intensify feelings toward him, and to try to talk directly about how they feel toward him and who he represents to them. He tries to notice when members are trying to "cross the river" and live in pieces of the Passionate Good Fit.

This leads to the work of doing and undoing. When members start trying out the Passionate Good Fit, they are committing a highly charged act of disloyalty. This act of disloyalty to the Passionate Bad Fit and its magnificence, shame, and excitement has enormous consequences for their identity, and their capacity for intimacy and attachment. Invariably, the members will be struck by how they suddenly feel cheated, that there are not the fireworks and the excitement as there was in the Passionate Bad Fit. They are angry, disillusioned, saddened, hurt, and furious with the process and with the therapist. They felt they were done in by my theory and my persuasiveness and power and command. The disillusion is massive and feels lethal to the therapist. Memories of their rages, and suppressed rages, are intensely present. Stories of being misled, of being severely disappointed, fill the group room. They are lonely, terrified, lost, and don't know who and where they are. They are unrecognizable.

> The member who constantly attempted to tell his parents that he was being abused by the day worker was left with his feeling that it was his job to clean up the mess. They refused multiple times to fire that worker. The group member still expects to be let down, to have to do it on his own, and to rarely trust any authority. This then made it much harder for him to be authoritarian when he needed it; instead, he tends to move into depression and hopelessness. He scrambles back to his old and powerful Passionate Bad Fit, which makes him feel more secure and safe there, with his appreciation of the enormous cost to his self-esteem and to his fear of risk-taking. His rage is presented more as passive resignation to his helplessness, willfulness, and hopelessness. He cannot let his spouse love him. He has gone back to his toxic early merged experience with the powerful mother who does not protect him, and he carries her shame to keep loving and protecting her from himself.

The therapist must listen, empathize, and take it in. The therapist has to take the heat here and allow the members to express their rage at their parents or at life, which they have never done. They have a glimpse of the injured infant, who could not utter these words to the world, of his body, and of his flawed parents. One member had to say, "It is not *my* fault." Another constructed a good mother inside herself to allow a lap and empathy during this time. Another member was able to see how she took care of her mother by staying home, not dating, not taking her sexuality seriously, and struggling with her weight.

They were all unable to have proper empathy for their plight. Instead, they blamed themselves for all they have lost again. They had made a vow to themselves that they were not going to try to merge again but live with who they were and enjoy the magnificence of their Passionate Bad Fit. The Passionate Bad Fit gets another shot of heroic imagery in being able to live, and endure, no matter what the cost. In reaction to all the internal conflicts and anxiety, there are stories of heroic acts by the others in the family.

> There is a father in the group who recounts his almost sadistic control of his son. He recounts it with the pride of a heroic act. Another patient, who has been quiet, finally cannot stand it and takes him on as the lousy father he is as well as the lousy self-centered father he had. He also has to acknowledge that the way he avoids being a lousy father is not to be a father at all. His use of loneliness and avoidance for him are his heroic acts. No one wants to hear that.

They undo the Passionate Good Fit and reclaim the shame and struggles of the Passionate Bad Fit, with a powerful sense of how magnificent it is that they have stayed loyal. This issue of loyalty vs. disloyalty is new and is rarely spoken of or taught at conferences or in the literature. It is crucial to allow the members to "cross over the river."

Stage VI: Doing and Undoing

The next step in the developmental model in this theory is coming to terms with their own Omnipotent Child and how they still live in the Passionate Bad Fit. They now can call other group members on their Omnipotent Child without being in danger that they will be asked to give up their own. They are able to acknowledge the internal structure, to give it up, with relationships outside of the group as well as with other group members.

> One man was finally able to forgive a woman because she did not fall in love with him, as he did with her. He had carried the grudge for over two years. He reluctantly was able to deal with his crushing disappointment with his mother. She did not medically take care of herself soon enough and died prematurely without the proper care. He loved her, he was her special one, the chosen one over his sister and his father. This chosen status was a powerful source of his shame, as well as carrying his mother's shame for all these years in his heroic style. He fought me tooth and nail over any interpretation I would make. He was opposed to psychiatrists, he refused to look for women rather than to live in a terrible Bad Fit relationship with the mother of his son. He would never find the right woman to replace the Passionate Bad Fit dance with his mother.

He found himself having many sexual and tender fantasies toward a woman in the group. She struggled with how difficult it was for her to accept love and be loved. She married a man who could not love her, and she struggled with leaving him or staying. They both could see the repetitions in their early life, and how magnificent their struggle was, which they said could not compare with the ordinariness of normal love and admiration. They were both trying to live in this Passionate Bad Fit, but both were weakening, and were starting to venture into the Passionate Good Fit, with tons of anxiety. He would disappear at times in the session, and she would cry easily, finally realizing that her tears were her sadness for what she never got, without the shame component. Without the shame, she said she could cry for the first time and feel it throughout her whole body and psyche. She felt free and alive, and maybe she could love. I told her that she could love, since I could feel her love for me. She smiled and cried some more, and said, "How hard it is to keep trying to live in loving you. Will the other members think I am foolish, or kill me, or make my life unsafe?"

While these connections are being made, I facilitate, and at the same time ask where I fit into this struggle. How do you feel toward me? Can you let yourself love me and have fantasies about me? Who am I for you at this point in our work?

One man finally starts to use my phrases in the group, and they remark that his battle with me seems to have ebbed. He wanted to be like me, but can he do it without shame? He recounted how ashamed he was when his parents got divorced. He hid from his friends and started to underperform in school. He became aware of how much his behavior with women, and toward himself, is related to the tremendous job he had of carrying the shame for both of his parents. His mother let herself die a medical death, and he carried her shame and his outrage and unforgiveness. His mother never apologized to him for dying the way she did. He demands that the woman apologize, apologize for not loving him the way he needed her to. To forgive the woman in the group was monumental for him. His shame was hidden by his grandiosity and his powerful struggles with justice and fairness. He admitted that he underachieved all his life, and wondered if the group thought that this affected his inability to get a second or third date on the matching services.

Stories of past regrets and past injuries, and the realization that they were profoundly affected by those events become the theme of the group meetings. They are trying to live in the Passionate Good Fit now, and as someone remarked, "Where are all the fireworks?" She is finally noticing that her husband loves her, and maybe she loves him. But where are the fireworks, as in "Bring in the Clowns" by Sondheim.

There is a member who lives in his reject button, which he earned from his parents acting as if he never made a difference in their lives. Underneath is an adorable little boy, who longs to be held and have a lap to claim as his own.

He re-created his family, his wife bringing in her grownup son, leaving him in third place. He struggled to let himself identify this, because his main goal is not to find a better life, but never to let go of his Passionate Bad Fit. He is married forever to his reject button, and the only time we do not see it or hear about it is when he can let himself be the adorable little boy. When he gets into his highly rigid, obsessive thinking in the group, I ask him, "What did you do to that adorable little boy? I prefer him to the adult you." The group agrees. He is usually confused by this and is only now beginning to show parts of the boy. He brings in funny cartoons and poetry sayings to the group, and talks of how much the group means to him. "This is the family I always wanted, and I love you all."

He usually will remind the group that his wife has insulted or hurt him, but she saved his life by getting him to an ER for his leg issues. He decides to investigate retirement homes and comes in excited with all promise and no rejection, then very quickly will undo this exciting, shameless experience that cannot be tolerated; there is no place for it in his internal life. He needs to undo and go back to being the loving husband who is in third place and feels rejected. The undoing is crucial to the final steps of moving into the Passionate Good Fit. I say, "You have to see how heroically you hold on to it, how much you give up to claim it, and how different your scary new world would be if you crossed over the river."

A woman who finally found, and let herself keep, the right man for herself goes back to see her aunt over the weekend. The aunt never wanted her to leave her for a man. She comes back to the group, triumphant and full of herself, as she tells us that "My aunt was right all the time, and this guy was just a terrible fantasy that only could lead to pain and disappointment." What a blow to all of us. We all thought we had made her healthy, and were enjoying our success when she tells us how she is no longer interested in that man. The group helps her withstand the loyalty to the aunt and how exciting it is to try to embrace the necessary disloyalty to the toxic wordless merger of infancy.

A guy finally meets the kind of woman he might be interested in, sees that woman, and at the same time will see his old girlfriend, whom he still deeply loves but she is unavailable. He gets furious with the group when we tell him to cancel the visit with his old love. I let him know that he is undoing his Passionate Bad Fit and its shameful grandiosity over the daily task of finding out more about this woman. It is a hard sell I have to make. The group, as it matures, remembers how they have gone through their own undoing, and really helps members to identify, expose, and stop the undoing.

This member is a good example of how I use my theory to switch the focus of the group's attention from one thing to another. The issue for him is the struggle he had about whether he would leave his wife and tolerate the loneliness he had before when he tried to find a woman. The group felt they were at an impasse with him. I suggested that the issue was not with his wife, but more with his tenacious hold on his heroically held rejection button. The involvement switched to an exploration of his Passionate Bad Fit, with the others trying to vocalize and name it. He was also letting us all know about the group's heroically held Passionate Bad Fits that they needed to attend to.

The painful awareness that life without shame feeding the grandiosity is very different than they ever expected. A melancholy hovers over the room as members keep getting angry at the world, at me, and at themselves for this duplicity. It is like the little 3-year-old child who suddenly gets scared when he has ventured too far away, feels untethered and lost, and runs back to his difficult mother and her lap. It is like the sorrow and hopelessness of little children when they have been disillusioned and terribly disappointed. There is no Santa Claus, there is no Easter Bunny, and we are splitting up and you will live with your dad and I will live here with your sister.

There are no fireworks in the lap. "Why do I need her lap, why aren't I strong enough, courageous enough and adventurist enough to not need the lap?" They begin to realize how they construct in fantasy, and in reality, the need to live in shame again to get back to the Passionate Bad Fit.

Stage VII: Sustaining the Passionate Good Fit Inside and Outside

This next phase is the realization that they must learn how to get rid of shame and acknowledge how they live in it and how they have disguised the shame. There is shame in shame.

An older member becomes slowly aware of his reluctance to be an authority and take a tough stance with his groups and with others. His Passionate Bad Fit is how long he can stay feeling less than, at the same time noticing how he gives up professional opportunities to be the powerful lawyer he wants to be. He will not take charge, even though it denies him further growth. His brilliance is a pain for him because it keeps making demands on him to excel, to expose his healthy narcissism and deal with the back and forth. He hides in his depression, his anxiety, and his fear of exposure. His narcissism is invested in being able to tolerate being harassed and traumatized and not have his parents rescue him. The rescue piece is relived through the myriad of treatments and therapists he sees to rescue him from his early captivity. The more he understands his depression and fears through living in the Passionate Bad Fit, the more he is willing to try more exposure of his narcissism and to notice that shame is too present in many of his thoughts and fantasies. His noticing the shame as a potential driver of the Passionate Bad Fit allows him to stand up to an older member and yell at him that he will no longer be insulted by him. The group applauds and he is stuck for the moment. Should he undo and bring up his anxiety and shame at yelling at this guy, or should he enjoy his outburst of healthy narcissism, not driven by shame? He is deciding, at this moment.

Gloria is another example of being caught up in the Passionate Bad Fit that would not allow her to choose a healthy mate or leave when she should leave. She grew up with parents who were children and acted as such, which in later years included too much drinking and less adult parenting. She was the special child of her father and would, in retrospect, try to be what he could not be. He fantasied that he was a brilliant academic scholar who was stuck with a middle-class company. Eventually she left home and traveled the world in risky adventures, to pursue her professional identity, as well as her father's dreams. There were many men on her travels, and she would get into triangles that always had the majesty of winning and the ignominy of losing. She then met a beautiful Hollywood-looking man who had his own boat and looked like a Midwestern hero like Paul Bunyan. He dazzled her, as did the boat trips together. But he was silent, unable to really notice her and communicate with her. I thought he was sadistic to her, about which she still fights me periodically. After 20 years of this depressing, humiliating marriage she made an appointment with me. She had heard that I could be tough, and I told her to leave him—which she immediately did, entered my group, and shortly thereafter met her present man, Jim. Her immediate acquiescence to my telling her to leave made me concerned about her relationship to authority figures, often denying her own power. She entered the group quietly, hidden in the shadows, and needed to be sought out before she would talk about anything. She was in hiding for a long time. I started to see her once weekly in individual therapy, which I did reluctantly but clearly could have done more.

I had faith in the group forces, but my narcissistic position changed over time, as did many things in my life: as the therapist, as well as the widowed, shocked 85-year-old man who suddenly realizes that he is vulnerable to everything. What a blow to my grandiosity! There I was trying to teach it, expose it, and help members explore it. At the same time, I was struggling with an infection that hospitalized me on and off for about a month. I held on to my healthy narcissism through the work in the group and through their love and care for me. This was spoken openly with the group, my admiration, and my love for how they cared for me, but now that I am healthy again, we need to talk about what it was like for them.

I know that many of you have had the job of taking care of a parent, or playing out their unconscious wishes, or protecting them, carrying their shame to be the special chosen child. What a mess this must have been for all of you.

They responded in many ways. I became the fallen, heroic idol of past wishes and illusions. They could live with it since I was telling them what it meant for me. Our parents rarely acknowledged our impact on them, except in a negative way. So where was their anger? They were surprised that they did not want to leave or see me die. They shamefully said they wanted me to live long enough so they could take my narcissism and use it for themselves. They felt they could be selfish, and I would understand and not retaliate. We all laughed and that relieved the tension in the group. Yes, we can all take from each other, since we are trying to live in each other as we were as infants with the symbiotic mother. We also seem to be learning the words for that wordless state of merged life. My illness allowed me to turn the event and feelings into the old issue of separation–individuation. Many members went back to those difficult times and began for the first time to appreciate how hard it was to leave safely the potentially toxic merger of infancy. They began to feel the losses and regrets in their life, for living in that merger and allowing it to be the source and energy for the Passionate Bad Fit.

> Gloria came alive when she noticed another woman in the group capturing my attention. From her hiding place, Gloria took her on, like no one else had. She shocked the group and herself. She was like the other woman in her triangles. She hated to lose and recalled how she would torment her sister, rather than deal with her parent's childlike behavior. We got glimpses of her strength, her risk-taking, and her willfulness. She always struggled with Jim's vulnerability, which tended to make her anxious, demanding, and angry. She struggled with the group and herself about staying with Jim. His childlike behavior drove her nuts. She was aware that she was living in the Passionate Bad Fit, which made her leave the family early, but also caused her to harass and hurt her sister. Both parents have died in the last 10 years. How do we move her from her Passionate Bad Fit when she knows she is in it, and prefers to struggle with her own anxiety than to leave him? He was able to love her in a way that no one had done. I gave her a suggestion many times that would allow her to figure out this dilemma without killing herself in the process. To my amazement, she refused in so many ways. She stonewalled me and the group. This all came to a head when she decided to purchase a special place that did demand Jim being able to care for her, due to its isolation. Now she had to truly evaluate his capacity to be an adult. This threw her into an intense state of anxiety and anger toward both herself and Jim.

It is not unusual, as group members, to know the Passionate Bad Fit and its grandiosity, and to structure situations that expose the Passionate Bad Fit for all of us to see. They cannot hide as they used to. There is relief in their coming out. Now the group can demand of each other that they name the Passionate Bad Fit in their lives. They ultimately agree to share it with everyone, and they unconsciously have merged with everyone and recreated a safer more loving merger than that of their wordless infancy. They have found the words they could never find before.

> Gloria tried to get Sam into therapy and settled for couple therapy. She would never take my suggestion. Finally, it became very clear to both of us that I was enacting her as a little girl and she was her mother and father, saying that they will not grow up. Her willfulness was awesome, as well as her pride in solving this problem without me. We had fiery exchanges about this, and she showed her contempt for me. I was able to express my outrage over her unwillingness to

even entertain my suggestion. This had given her an excellent opportunity to be as contemptuous of me as she had been of her parents, her first husband, and Jim, as well as herself. I acknowledged how proud I was for her to take me on, and to let us see these other well-hidden parts of herself: her contempt, her willfulness, and her need to be heroically unappreciated. The group saw this as an impasse with them, as to whether she would leave Jim and follow my suggestion. I said it was a stalemate within herself, when or if she gives up and move on from her Passionate Bad Fit or persists in this exciting, grandiose, messy, toxic merger with her childlike parents. She loved defeating me, as she was trying to defeat her grandiosity and not notice how scared she was that Jim could or would be capable of really taking care of her. If she could not defeat her own Passionate Bad Fit, then maybe she could make me be that part of her: the small, vulnerable, and helpless little girl up against her parents. We both worked a great deal on the intimacy between us. She was able to hear for the first time her own rage and frustration as I shared with her how difficult it was to get her to listen and act accordingly. "How hard that must have been for you as a kid. No wonder you belted around your sister. You did not want to kill your parents. But you let yourself be battered round in that 20-year relationship that finally ended."

And to this day she cannot see him as sadistic. It has been hard for us to get her to notice sadism and masochism in this relationship with Jim. She is more struck by the excitement of it all, as well as shame starting to sneak in. This shame is the fuel that keeps the Passionate Bad Fit running all the time, and it will not allow a chance for healthy narcissism to flourish. The shame you carry for your parents. The shame of refusing to grow up, and not noticing what was happening in their family and you. When the shame is revealed and accepted, we are on the way to allow a shift from living in the Passionate Bad Fit and taking the risk of trying out the Passionate Good Fit. We then have to decide what to do with the shame.

Empathy comes in here, as very few of these members have a great deal of empathy for themselves. They have it for their parents, but not for themselves. The empathy cuts into the hidden shame and the Passionate Bad Fit is weakened by this, and the chance for escape to the Passionate Good Fit is now more possible. They are more able to take a risk and cross over the river.

Stage VIII: Leaving and Acknowledging the Risks and How Different Life Is without Shame as the Organizer and Driver

This ultimate phase is partly didactic and partly experiential. The group is well aware of the need to undo their gains, and they need help in trying to ward off this undoing.

Ginger tells us how she has crossed the river in so many ways, but gets tormented by fantasies of tornados, or nuclear war that will destroy all her gains and her loved animals. For the first time, she is able to feel that she likes where she works, enjoys the responsibility she is thriving on, and, for the first time, feels like she can come to peace with her younger brother. She can enjoy her power, her competence, her mind, and now her capacity to love and be close to people. She is not pushing people away as she did; she is now welcoming her friends differently, as she now welcomes the group as a friendly family that will help her be more comfortable with her womanhood. She had a dream of carrying home a large, oversized bag from a trip that was filled with her clothes. She was curious about the big valise. The group was able to tell her it was her unused vagina, which is now open and welcoming. She was shocked but thrilled at the same time.

She started the ball rolling by asking, "How can we make sure that we cannot undo?" The group shifted to some teaching on my part about the need for radar inside. I said, "You need something that will tell you that you are in dangerous territory. The radar should be connected to your body in some way, so the body, which carries all your history and the Passionate Bad Fit, can let you thwart this inevitable move toward the Passionate Bad Fit again." The group explores various attempts and techniques of building radar systems. One person says that when she begins to feel euphoric, she knows there will be a shift down to despair. "The euphoria is my radar to stop the undoing as best I can." Another says that when she begins to feel inferior to her brother and his millions, she is in the process of undoing. Another notices that when she actually feels happy, undoing is around the corner. Now, when she can feel happy and use it as radar, it helps her to not give up the happiness and instead try to sustain it. She can learn to live with it and build muscles to sustain and hold it as her own and not give it up. Another wonders if, when he needs to remind himself how he did not make millions in his business, he is trying to undo the fact that he and his family are in great shape for whatever they want and need. Another member always wondered why she still wants to sit down with her mother and have a heart-to-heart talk. That is her radar to let her know that she is getting uncomfortable with a healthy life and healthy narcissism, and it is time to undo it and feel those bells and whistles and fireworks again.

There are so many different ways to build radar, and I feel it must be done as part of their maturing and leaving the treatment as a healthy, mature, evolved person. They can then say goodbye to each other and hold the new growth, locking it up in a toolbox filled with all new goodies for their use. The goodbye is without shame, filled with tears and love and gratitude and joy and good wishes, and how they hope someday to recreate for themselves this family of caring and talk and love and respect and mutuality and living inside each other and separating when ready.

Chapter 3

The Omnipotent Child Syndrome

The Role of Passionately Held Bad Fits in the Formation of Identity

I am extending here the works of Durkin and Glatzer (1997) and Kauff (1997), in their elucidating the role of transference and regression in mobilizing affect to moderate and alter character pathology in analytic group psychotherapy. This chapter takes *passion* as its cardinal affect. Passion is defined here as a powerful somatic emotion such as love, excitement, arousal, hate, or anger. The patient's and the group's passion is expressive of, and indicative of, its earliest good and bad fits, both within the history of the group and the history of the individual members and therapists. In the group process, individuals recreate the bad fits through multiple attachments to other members of the group. The individual patient's and the group's life are suffused with these Passionate Bad Fit attachments. The working-through process then takes on an urgency of its own. This urgency becomes a healthy part of the analytical culture of the group and persists throughout the history of the group, regardless of the members present.

The Omnipotent Child is a construct to help therapists conceptualize and treat the origins of these highly resistant narcissistic islands of identity that plague the patient, and interfere in the development of a full, mature life. It is that part of the internal psychic structure that is the final common pathway of all the passionately held bad fits that characterize not only the person's object ties and attachments but also his most powerful internal psychic identity. The "omnipotence" referred to here is different from the more common usage, as in the omnipotence of a small child's magical thinking, or the grandiosity of a narcissistic defense, or an adolescent's inflated view of himself. It refers instead to the power of an early fixed, somatically driven, island of identity. It feels to the patient as if it is indestructible, tenacious, and all-powerful over important aspects of the person's choices as to attachments and issues of mutuality and intimacy. The omnipotence also refers to its demand to be highly idealized and held tightly with extreme loyalty. At times, this loyalty is heroic, to the point of giving up one's normal and healthy passions for the passion of the bad fit. The source for the Passionate Bad Fit rests in the earliest attachment experiences that are mediated through the central nervous system, particularly the sensory somatic apparatus. These early sensory somatic experiences affect the laying down of brain structure and potentially set into motion the internal representations of the attachment experiences, both healthy and unhealthy.

DOI: 10.4324/9781032705835-4

The concept of the Omnipotent Child hinges on the attachment to these internalized infantile passions that know no bounds in their claims on self and others. The earlier the bad fit, the more profound effect it will have on character pathology. This is further complicated by the pre-verbal bad fit and is then only left to the repetitive need to recreate those passionate bodily states, as well as the need to attempt to put into some symbolic representation those early experiences (Chuah, 1986).

The Omnipotent Child Syndrome is a cluster of emotionally driven behaviors and attachment style patterns that are identifiable in a certain group of patients. They are high-functioning, highly likable, with sophisticated insight, yet are plagued by chronically unhealthy attachments. Despite the unhappy, unfulfilling nature of these relationships, people remain in them. Characteristically, they are stable, long standing, relatively non-chaotic, and tend not to incur their partner's wrath and abandonment. These patients can be characterized by their failure to respond to different and multiple therapeutic modalities, yet they continue to search for treatment. In treatment, they tend to be model patients, being well behaved, with little acting out. They tend to stay in therapy for long periods of time, yet rarely stir up anxiety in the group and the therapist. The therapist tends to be lulled into a state of benign satisfaction, not noticing that little basic character change is made. The patient, with the therapist's blessing, then leaves therapy, only soon to search for another. Therapists are clearly seeing more of these chronic, treatment-resistant patients. Multiple theories and techniques have been constructed to deal with this population, without recognizing the uniqueness of this syndrome (Alonso & Rutan, 1993; Gans & Alonso, 1998; Leszcz, 1989; Roller & Nelson, 1999; Schlachet, 1998; Stone & Gustafson, 1982; Wright, 1998).

The good fit, in which the child's needs are met in a good enough way, allows the earliest primary dyad to grow together, to heal, to know the internal mental states of each other, and to be mutually soothed. This neutralizes aggression in both the body and the internal developing psyche and allows for healthy growth to occur in order to take on the next life challenge. The good fit leads to a sense of optimism about life, and the body is experienced as a healer and source of constancy. It leads to a potential for creativity, and a sense of being able to be excited, joyful, and full of pleasure. Most importantly, the good fit leads to a need for other good fits. Hence, the chance of picking an appropriate mate is much higher. The good fit is akin to the secure attachment that is crucial for "reflective functioning" that enables children to conceive of other's beliefs, feelings, attitudes, desires, hopes, knowledge, imagination, pretense, and plans. This ability to be curious and explore the other's actions and their meanings contributes powerfully to affect regulation and impulse control, and self-monitoring (Fonagy, 1999). I propose that when the psychological states of the mothering figure do not fit the developing infant's needs and innate constitution, deep and long-lasting object relations effects are embedded in the body ego of the infant, affecting all further self and/or character development. These bad fits lead to uncertainty, shame, a lack of constancy, un-neutralized aggression, negativity about all future choices, and a flourishing of attendant narcissistic defenses and structures that become embedded in both the individual and the couple. This is akin to the insecure attachment that renders the child unable to regulate his internal and external world and lacks reflective functions Lichtenberg (1999). This unregulated state of being reflects a lack of containment of the aversive affective states in the child as well as in the dyad.

These uncontained aversive and passionate affective states, i.e., aggression, anxiety, and somatic arousal are, in fact, contained in a paradigm that I call the Omnipotent Child. Its function is to sustain old bad fits that fix, and hold, one's idea of one's self, or identity, in an intimate relationship. This fixing of one's idea of one's self stabilizes the child's sense of self, albeit in an unhealthy stable identity. It is the agent that disdains change and growth and that prefers the sameness and consistency of the earliest, highly somatic, and affectively passionate intimate moments in their life. It is their anchor in a churning sea. This paradigm echoes the work of Stolorow and Lachman (1980) and Cohen (2000), who redefine narcissistic character traits and behaviors as that system of beliefs that serve to stabilize the sense of self (identity) in face of all realities, object relationships, and fantasies. My hypothesis is that passionate early somatic experiences coalesce within the psyche to shape profound early ideas of one's self that define the moments of intimacy in relationships.

The Neurobiological and Attachment Bases for the Omnipotent Child

The infant at birth is now thought to be prewired for perceptual awareness and is not a blank screen as was thought earlier (Beebe, Lachman, & Jaffe, 1997; Stern, 1985). This prewiring helps the infant develop attentional ties to part-objects such as the mouth, the eyes, and the voice, which are all expressions of the mothering figure. It is then thought that these early part-object experiences are fostered and augmented by stimulus-seeking behavior, rather than only by tension-reducing experiences. There are multiple observations of infants showing that, when they are somatically challenged, they will increase their stimulus-seeking behavior. Stern argues that the infant needs as much stimulation as he does tension reduction and postulates that when the body is not stimulated enough, it will seek stimulation, while if the stimulation is too high, it will move toward tension reduction.

Stern makes a distinction between the physiological needs and the psychobiological needs of the infant. The psychobiological needs that stimulus-seeking mutual behavior pertains to are mediated through the early attachment processes in the infant's experience. Freedman (1989) postulates that the following conflict-free psychobiological needs form the basis for the infant's core identity. These needs are curiosity, excitement, sense of self, self-differentiation, the self's view of the body as either enemy or ally, and the sense of self as either good, calm, and contained, or disorganized, disruptive, and inconstant. These core somatically influenced identities can be adaptive or maladaptive. They become modes of functioning and templates for later intimate affective states and develop into character traits that are experienced as truly one's self.

Pine (1985) tries to integrate the psychoanalytic positions of Mahler (1968) with the object relationists and the new child/infant observations previously mentioned. Pine emphasizes the powerful influence of "moments" in an infant's life, as well as the critical nature of the role of the quiet pleasure time for the infant to self-regulate, and to develop object constancy. Pine amplifies that the influential "moments" in an infant's developmental life are the points associated with high-intensity bodily sensation and high-intensity object relations. As such, they have a psychological significance far beyond what can be measured by their temporal duration. All these developmental "moments" elicit, with the same intensity, bad fits and good fits that endure.

The newest research in neurobiology emphasizes the role of somatic sensations as crucial for laying down neuronal connections in the brain. Kandel (1998) states that, in simple animals, experience produces sustained changes in the effectiveness of neural connections by altering gene expression. Everyday sensory experience, sensory deprivation, and learning can lead to weakening or strengthening of synaptic connections. This recent evidence clearly supports that such experience produces sustained neuronal changes that have a lasting effect. Kandel goes so far as to state that this distinctive modification of the brain architecture, along with a unique genetic makeup, constitutes the biological basis for individuality.

Where Does the Omnipotent Child Fit into the Schema of the Early Infant's Life?

The Omnipotent Child is laid down in the internalized part-objects that are the hallmark of the body ego, and hence are a part of the internal psychic structure of the emerging child. These early introjects of part-objects, and the autonomous ego functions that are prewired and constitutional for that infant, will become embedded and constitute an important part of the identity of the infant. The embedding occurs at the "moments" referred to earlier. When there is a high-intensity somatic experience, coupled with an equally high-intensity object relation, the internal body ego becomes suffused with a Passionate Good or Bad Fit. The passion describes the high intensity that is needed to cathect the introject and to embed it. It also describes the somatic arousal generated by this fit. These fits, which are not too dissimilar to the molding and laying down of the brain architecture that Kandel speaks of, I postulate, become the source of the child's core identity and foreshadow his or her relationships with others and with the self. How the child regulates its body shapes and heavily influences its sense of goodness, badness, competence, and incompetence. Elvin Semrad stated on grand rounds,

> The first object you love or hate is your own body. You love it when it feels good and hate it when it feels bad. It feels good when it's held and bad when it's causing pain. When we hurt we hold ourselves, don't we?
>
> (Rako & Mazer, 1983)

These early fits also, most importantly, influence the shaping of how intimacy between the self and others is laid down and experienced in the body and then in the internal life.

The Omnipotent Child in Group Therapy

How is the patient's Omnipotent Child experienced and expressed in the group? The Omnipotent Child is best explored in the group setting, as there are multiple choices of attachments for it to be played out with, and the very nature of the group is to form attachments. The group's infectious and regressive proclivities allow the group members to move to the earliest infantile and preverbal experiences more quickly. These powerful group drives encourage both the fleshing out of the Omnipotent Child as well as the group's defense against it. The collective unconscious Omnipotent Child in the patients serves to unite the patients in a highly intimate and passionate way. It leads to group cohesion, yet, in a malignant way, it can be the reservoir for future group resistances, stalemates, and repetitive behaviors that don't move the group forward. In this context, it is also possible for a group member to find someone in the group who feels safe, while the Passionate Bad Fit is explored with another member. The Omnipotent Child longs for someone to know him and to be attached yet, at the same time, actively rejects any attempts to be loved and understood. Unlike the narcissistic character, the Omnipotent Child stirs up empathy and warmth in the therapist and group members, rather than contempt and disdain. His injuries and pain are present along with his pleasant imperiousness, but his affective states are not nearly as obnoxious as the expression of the usual narcissistic entitlements. The Omnipotent Child sadly, and warmly, exclaims his struggle about being stuck in his dilemma and with his ambivalence in accepting and rejecting help. He is ashamed of his position, yet feels heroically glued to it, and feels no one can help him disentangle himself. His need to reject help comes from his passionate fear of losing his identity. That leaves him stuck in a sad, poignant, lonely hold on intimate isolation. He loves and trusts his Omnipotent Child more than anyone else. He engenders warmth and love in others in the group. However, eventually they will be disappointed, aroused, and frustrated, as he was at various points in his development. He will acknowledge his Omnipotent Child and laugh with others about it but will defend it as if he has no other resources. He can feel and act like a loveable, sad, despairing, excited, temper-tantrum-throwing two-year-old.

After lengthy periods of time, these patients, with their Omnipotent Child, wear down the therapist and group members by their stubborn, tantrum-like quality of holding onto positions they know and articulate are irrational and absurd. However, unlike the narcissistic and borderline character disorders, they usually do not engender hateful feelings. This stubborn part of the patient is persistent and powerful in his warm rejection of others and in his own state of internal idealization. The Omnipotent Child is highly valued, since it was that part of the child that kept the attachments alive, gave stability to an inherently unstable environment, and organized the internal and external passions in their environments. This part of the ego is highly loved and admired, yet its function is to keep alive the old, unhealthy passionate attachments. Patients love their Omnipotent Child and think and feel about it as the most exciting thing in their lives. It is the source and reservoir for their passion. Seeing this syndrome allows the therapist and the group to analyze these defenses in a different way. It goes beyond the view of defenses against fears of dissolution, as in the Kohutian formulations of self psychologists, and instead, focuses on the excitement inherent in the holding onto these unrealistic and unhealthy parts of the person's identity and behaviors. The therapist can make group-as-a-whole interventions with respect to the group's collusion to keep the Omnipotent Child hidden and all-powerful, or they could try to tolerate the anxiety of being without this early identity and rely on each other to be held until they have worked through it.

> Mary complains endlessly in the group about how her husband, and the world, keep disappointing her, and brings in one example after another. The therapist and the group inform her that the issue isn't her husband and the world, or the group, but the intense excitement and power she feels to be organized and have her identity expressed in her disappointments. She has to choose between this old identity and tolerating the fear of being organized around not being disappointed. Can anything compare with the excitement of her next disappointment? Who will do her in, and how will they do it? What great moments she lives in; how spectacular her life is. She's built a monument to the excitement of her earliest disappointments in her life.

These patients can go for years without giving into their needs for nurturance, love, and healthy passion. This is their heroic loyalty. Why else would they love and identify with the worst parts of their parents and families, except as a way to hold on to their bad fit attachments and hence their identity. For the most part, the Omnipotent Child is connected to people, but the relationships are seductively frustrating and arousing in that they promise so much and give so little. Their ability to seduce and frustrate is their recreation of the earliest bad fits but also plays out the aggression in the Omnipotent Child. The Omnipotent Child trusts enough to stay in the group for prolonged periods of time, unlike the narcissistic character disorder. In fact, the full emergence and acknowledgment of the Omnipotent Child in the patient really doesn't happen until many other issues are dealt with, and the resolution of the patient's Omnipotent Child usually signals the beginning of the end of the treatment process.

In the group, to allow the development and resolution of the Omnipotent Child, I encourage the new and old members' overt transference reactions to each other and to me, as soon as they can tolerate it. I also encourage their attention to all bodily sensations and physical and fantasy desires to facilitate perception of their part-object attachments and to deepen therapeutic regression as they develop Omnipotent Child feelings and bad fits in the group process. I encourage the members to try to recreate in their imagination and to put into words or pictures their first year of life. Even though, at the beginning, the therapist takes center stage, as the group moves on developmentally the therapist and the group work together in analysis by the group and for the group. Over time, in the group situation, one can see quite clearly the influence of the good and bad fits on the choice of object, as well as on the course of the relationship. Implicit in the group model is the assumption that there are periodic regressions to earlier phases of development that are experienced and defended by all in the group. As the group dynamic permits more regression and exploration of the individual's internal structures, as well as his capacity for object ties, the telescopic view of the origins of the bad fits comes into focus and gets played out in the group, at each developmental stage. The group offers patients an opportunity to re-explore the original bad fits and injuries, and the group has a chance to respond differently. Through repeated experiences, where the patient's Omnipotent Child is in full view, the group's reflective function (Fonagy, 1999) aids the patient and the whole group to develop a different relationship with this part of themselves and in their group relationships. Through these repeated group rapprochement experiences, as well as individual moments of memories, fantasies, and dreams, members can attempt to picture and put into words their idea of their first year of life. As a result, the bad fits will soften and allow some good fits to intervene. Hence, some of the constitutional and relational aggression and anxiety will be neutralized. When the therapist or group members attempt to tackle these bad fits, rageful, and/or depressed storms occur because the patients experience these attempts as intrusions, leaving them bereft of their identity. Many patients at this moment say, "Who am I without this way of being?" At these moments, the therapist emphasizes that what is at stake here is not just behavior or moods, but the patient's very identity. It is as if patients feel like they have lost everything, are nothing, and have stepped over a cliff into the unknown. They describe feeling like they are without their skin, or they can't be held or touched because their skin is too sunburned, or they have a "hairball" inside that has to come up and can't be extruded. It is reassuring to the patient when the therapist and other group members let him know that he will be "held" as long as he needs to be. The patient and the group will then feel confident to venture out of the dark, chasm-like, unknown space, with the beginnings of a new identity and new ways of attaching to self and others. In my experience, the group process is the best place for a patient to be held in the terrifying anxiety of a loss of body identity until they emerge on the other side.

Case Examples that Illustrate and Demonstrate the Omnipotent Child in the Group

Bob is a 40-year-old single man who, prior to joining my twice-weekly group five years ago, had been in treatment on and off for the last twenty years. His story was one of chronic, intermittent depression that had been resistant to all previous treatments. His depression seemed to start in college after a major disappointment with a girl. The group perceived him as a sad, adorable little boy who needed to be loved, encouraged, and tolerated. Rarely has he been confronted with his negativism, pessimism, and his constant devaluing of the group process. The task with Bob and the group, after working through early conflicts, was to identify his Omnipotent Child. Through repeated examples of the nature of his attachment to the group and to himself, he produced a dream that symbolized his Omnipotent Child and gave the group a chance to identify and work with this material. His dream was that he had just scored the winning touchdown for his high-school team, and was totally relieved when he realized that he had broken his leg on the play. He would never score another touchdown, he said proudly to the group as he related this pivotal dream. The smile on his face was infectious, as was his body language, as he sat more upright than usual, and was more excited and spontaneous. His moodiness and sullenness were gone. The whole group laughed and joked with him and found the dream exciting. He had seduced and charmed the group with his bald statement of his Omnipotent Child. The therapist then pursued, over time, the group's collusion with Bob to maintain the status quo of his Omnipotent Child. A woman in the group said for the first time that Bob really gave her nothing and she felt starved by him. Another man felt more courageous to speak up about how he understood and identified with Bob's position of never wanting to satisfy anyone.

Bob, who was the track and football star on his high-school team, was tired of being the star, and decided in college that he wouldn't be that anymore. He acknowledged that he was overvalued by his mother for the first two years of his life, which ended rather abruptly with the birth of his brother. He thought that the women in the world should love his depression and moodiness and ambivalence as much as he did. Later in the group work, as the denial was eroded and he was comfortable exploring the passion embedded in his bad fits, he revealed that his body always felt that it was too easily stimulated. He reluctantly revealed that, at times, he felt flooded by his mother's over-involvement. In the past, he tried to calm himself and his body through drugs and then ultimately through depression and sullenness. The group process was a continuous threat of being too physically stimulating and arousing. His Omnipotent Child organized around his need to keep his body quiescent and protect him from being too stimulated. He was passionately on alert and would not let much get through, but it left him isolated and unable to tolerate normal and healthy arousal in relationships. His Omnipotent Child was embedded in the overvaluation in the first years of life, which coincided with intense somatic experiences that were either constitutionally determined and/or related to the mutually exciting idealizing relationship with his mother.

Joyce was a highly valued member of her twice-weekly group for many years, even though she could be quite sarcastic toward members of the group, as well as overwhelming in her pressured speech patterns and in her anxiety. She had been either compliant or angry and dismissive of the other group members. The group sensed an underlying fragility in her, and was quite supportive of her, even in her attacks. They saw these attacks as her "street smarts" that they envied. The group members conspired for their own reasons in a group defense of her and the group's Omnipotent Child. She would tell someone who recently discussed a loss to "get over it." She told a man who was struggling with his effectiveness with his wife to stop being a chicken and a wimp. She told others at various times to stop whining and shape up and give her something to work with. She was tactless and demanding, yet she avoided the group's rage and open hostility. She threatened to leave the group when I didn't personally inform her of my return from a medical absence, even though her husband had been notified, and there was a message to that effect on my answering machine. She exhibited exquisite sensitivity to being "left out," yet was impatient and insensitive to other's expression of neediness. Her Omnipotent Child resided in the passionate position of being 'left out." When Joyce's mother was four months pregnant with Joyce, her two-year old son died suddenly. The family never discussed the death of this child. There were no pictures of him, and she only found out about his existence when she was 20 years old. She had to compete with a ghost all her life, and never understood why she couldn't capture mother's undivided attention. Her very early identity was formed around being left out and not part of mother's internal life. This early relationship with her mother was most likely felt in her skin and her body and in her desperate, pressured, speech pattern that, at times, overwhelmed the group. She never could get in, and she has spent the rest of her life either feeling hurt about being left out or getting people to feel left out.

A new member, Resa, entered the group. Her issues were her agonized conflict over her wish to be taken care of by her damaged, unreliable, and angry mother (the therapist) versus her need to be in the exciting, arousing middle of two fighting parents. In one session, Resa was imploring the therapist-mother to help her deal with a fight she had on her hands at work. Resa ignored the group and directed everything at the therapist. Joyce finally said to Resa, "Get over it." Resa exploded at Joyce and called her toxic. She raged at Joyce and said that she could not stand her arrogance, her dismissiveness of the other group members, her callousness, and, most of all, the group's collusion with her about this. Joyce was devastated by Resa's comments. Buddy, who had watched his mother and sister fight all his life, finally cried and said he couldn't stand this fight. It scared him so much. Joyce threatened again to leave the group. The therapist said that this fight might be about whether the group could or couldn't tolerate the exposure of the Omnipotent Child in both Resa and Joyce. Joyce couldn't tolerate Resa's attachment to me, and her longings for it conflicted with her Omnipotent Child's position of being alone, angry, unloved, and left out. Resa needed to appreciate that her intense need to be the agonized, excited arbiter of intense and crucial fights was her Omnipotent Child. Buddy needed to recognize that his Omnipotent Child was that he was going to be the best little girl/little boy that he and his mother and sister would forever, mutually admire. Seeing the women in the group fight reminded Buddy how ineffective he felt and still feels in claiming his manhood from the fighting and seductive women. Each of these members, and the rest of the group, then struggled for months until they could appreciate and discuss that what was really toxic was their attachment to their Omnipotent Child and their collusion with each other to keep that hidden.

In this case, and in many other group situations, the group members and the therapist collude in not starting any rageful storms within it. The group members want to live with their passionate old restrictive identities and prefer not to have them intruded upon. New members, like Resa, serve a real purpose in upsetting the apple cart. The passion in each of the members in the above-cited group "moments" could be seen by the agitation in the members' bodies, their tears, their rage, and their abject terror. Joyce was able, after a period of time, to trace her early years with her profound identity of being left out. She could then finally ask the therapist questions about his personal life, and show some empathy toward him about events that occurred in his life. Finally, she could ask her mother about the dead child, and know how his death affected her and all her relationships. She began to be softer with her husband and the group. Her tears are now about her losses and her regrets about how she led her life. It is a painful path toward incorporating her new identity.

This case will illustrate how the early preverbal bad fits, which give rise to attendant somatic sensations, plagued this patient all his life.

Jim, a 38-year-old single man, has noticed that he is still anxious and suspicious of the therapist and the group, even though he has worked with us for the last 6 years in a twice-weekly group. He has changed enormously in this time, but his sense of apprehension, distrust, and irritability lingers. He can still experience the therapist as his sadistic father, and see the group as his passive mother who didn't protect him. As the group was engaged in exploring their first year of life through fantasy, imagination, bodily sensations, and their recollection of their first year in this group, Jim was able, for the first time, to relate his early childhood experiences. His first year of childhood was marked by many disruptive moments. His father was jealous of and apparently angry at his closeness to his mother. His parents built an addition to the house, then sold it and moved to another home when he was 6 months old. His mother was pregnant with his younger brother when he was 4 months old. His reflections on his fantasy of his earliest moments had to do with taking in as much stimulation as he could tolerate and suffering in silence. His body was exposed to loud noises, chaos, and intense parental anxiety, which influenced the normative caring experiences of childhood. He imagined his mother was nervous and unsure of herself when he was an infant. He felt that she could barely manage him, with her husband's intense demands and her need to focus on the baby inside of her. His father's sadism and his mother's anxiety about containing his father reinforced these early bad fits. She felt that she was unable to protect her son. His body and self grew up in an unsafe household. His early exploration of his body and his genitals usually involved self-inflicted, eroticized pain. His Omnipotent Child, as defined by the group, was that part of him that could only live in a highly threatening, exciting, dangerous situation. All other relationships felt dull and boring. It manifested itself in the group by his sadistically teasing and taunting the group through his physically dangerous relationship with his live-in partner. One could see his big grin as he taunted the group. The group eventually labeled his grin as that "shit-eating grin." At no time did anyone get furious with him. Instead, they empathized and suffered with him. They did express frustration, but not the rage and anger they felt at another member of the group, who was a narcissistic character who wouldn't attach to the group in a way that felt meaningful and alive to them.

The therapist commented at times about the group's helplessness in trying to get Jim to leave his partner, but didn't he really express for the group each member's difficulty and arrogance in holding on to their own Omnipotent Child? After the conflicts with his father and mother were resolving, he was able to talk about the chronic anxiety that suffused his body and mind. He was finally able to lose weight with the help of the group's suggestions. His later work in the group was to shift this basic body identity to one of safety, trust, and respect. He no longer threatens himself or the group, and has become my "co-therapist" in the group. As the arrogantly held position of the early bad fit diminished, for something better in the group, he began to experience sadness, and a different form of anxiety. This anxiety reflected the unknown space that must be crossed, to move into and embrace the new identity not based on the intimacy of the Omnipotent Child.

In the three previous cases, the shift from an old identity to a new identity, and hence new behavior, is explored. A new sense of intimacy is accomplished in the group by the therapist's, and then the group's, insistence that the patients look at, examine, and explore, the passion connected to the old bad fit, and thus the Omnipotent Child is identified. Through examining the passion of these early bad fits, the patient and the group are then able to experience it in their intimacies in the group, as well as to begin to recall the earlier moments in their life, that were exhilarating, frightening, overstimulating, or deadening. This exploration also reworks for the group their concepts and ideas of the first year of their lives, and how the preverbal experiences are still manifest in the group and in their lives. A great deal of emphasis is given to the attempts to put into words, pictures, fantasies, or dreams, those early intimate moments in the first year that led to the passion of the bad fit.

The exploration of the passion in the Omnipotent Child helps the group members to short-circuit their own defenses. Patients have said, at various times, that the concept of the Omnipotent Child helped them understand, without shame, their struggle with relationships. The concept of the Omnipotent Child helps patients understand their imagined inherent badness for failing to live in a good fit, and for not understanding the impact of that first year of life. The group is then better able to appreciate the power of this passion and its repetitive nature, and its ultimate impact on their identity and their most intimate relationships. The therapist can now, along with the group, better empathize with their impossibly stuck position of wanting to give up that part of themselves that has been the repository of the most passionate and exciting moments in their life. How and why would anyone give that up for ordinary daily life experiences? Why would they find passion in relationships built on mutuality, trust, and respect, and what kind of passion could match the passion of the early bad fits?

Embedded in all relationships is the opportunity to rework old internal issues and conflicts or be doomed to repeat them. The need for intimacy and its demands on the relationship, and the intrapsychic and somatic parts of the individuals involved, set in motion the older developmental cycles that were experienced in infancy and later developmental milestones. Within each phase of the developmental cycle, there is the potential for a good or a bad fit, which defines the proclivities and vulnerabilities of the developing self-identity and parameters of the relationships that are forming, and are formed. The good or bad fit is determined by the special moments when the child's needs must be met by the mothering figure, who is either ready or not ready, internally or externally, to meet those demands. Fred Pine (1994) states when the "child's moment meets the mother's character or conflicts a magnification of the moment is likely to take place" (p. 20).

The magnification that Pine talks about here is the very nidus on which the good and bad fits are laid down. These are the crystallization points for these good fits. Each major phase of development such as latency, adolescence, college years, work, marriage, loss, birth of children, falling in love, falling out of love, dealing with disappointments, and learning to live with success are demands on both the psyche and the body to regress to the earliest phases of development. Therefore, each step in a person's life gives a telescopic view into the earliest phases and how they were settled, as well as how any previous damage continues into each subsequent life challenge.

Summary

The Omnipotent Child is present in all of us, as we all have had, at various times, bad fits that have shaped our character formation, as seen and as experienced in intimate situations and relationships. The degree of passion of the Omnipotent Child depends on the degree, timing, repetitiveness, and nature of the bad fit. It is also highly subject to constitutional givens around the somatic sensitivities in each person, and especially in the early dyadic relationships of the first years of life. Once the bad fit is embedded, the person keeps seeking out other bad fit relationships, to keep alive his passionate identity. The Omnipotent Child is treatable, since it yearns for attachments and will tolerate the frustration of intense group treatment. In the presence of a soothing and mutually beneficial rapprochement phase, which allows for a correction from a bad fit to a good enough good fit, it can ultimately succumb. The notion that there could be something better is experienced. That something better is the newfound group attachments and passions that now consist of pleasure, joy, and excitement, without shame and humiliation.

The Omnipotent Child Syndrome is an attempt to integrate the newer versions of the role narcissistic behaviors play in the stabilizing of identity with the relationists' point of view (Schermer, 2000). It is the concealed passion of these early fits that embeds and keeps alive the narcissistic bad fits, which shapes the structure of intimacies in relationships. When the group can put into words or pictures the earliest preverbal experiences, then there is a chance for a new internal structure to form that is based on healthy passions such as mutuality, trust, respect, and attraction.

Acknowledgment

Reprinted from the *International Journal of Group Psychotherapy*, 52(1) 67–87 © 2002 The American Group Psychotherapy Association, Inc. Reprinted by permission of Taylor & Francis Ltd. (http://www.tandfonline.com) on behalf of The American Group Psychotherapy Association, Inc.

Chapter 4

How the Passionate Bad Fit and Omnipotent Child Develop

Your way of being in an intimate relationship is founded in your earliest ways of relating with your primary caregiver. The baby must be nurtured. Simply put, good fits occur when the earliest experiences of infancy, between mother and infant, are mutually satisfying. Does the mother know what the baby needs? Does she know how to soothe the baby? Does she allow the baby to, at times, turn away from her? Does she allow the baby to express and meet its own needs? The baby, by expressing its needs, will show some of its innate wiring and makeup. Can the mother regulate both her own internal needs and the child's internal needs, so that both mother and child feel attached to one another in a healthy way? They can both feel satisfied. The healthier the mothering figure, the easier and more natural these tasks of early mothering become. The better the attachment is, the better the baby will develop.

When the infant must rely on nurturing from a difficult, unsatisfying, under- or over-stimulating mother, the infant, to get his needs met, must adapt to the mother's needs. To avoid abandonment, the baby tries to help the mother not feel too bad about her mothering. In these situations, the baby must fit into the mother's needs more than his own. A conflict arises. This is the Bad Fit. And this is where the Omnipotent Child has its beginnings as the container for the Bad Fits. The Bad Fit results in uncontained passionate affective states, such as aggression, anxiety, and somatic arousal. These affective states, if not contained, can cause internal chaos. The Omnipotent Child serves to contain the Bad Fits. Though necessary to preserve a sense of stability, the cost of this containment is high. It cements one's idea of oneself in an unhealthy identity. It works to preserve these earliest Bad Fits. It stabilizes the Bad Fit identity, which then makes it difficult to change. The Omnipotent Child, in its powerful way, fixes and holds one's idea of oneself and one's identity in an intimate relationship.

For example, when after a good feeding the baby is resting, but the mother wants to play with the baby, the baby responds by turning away and perhaps crying (Beebe, Lachman, & Jaffe, 1997). If the mother continues to approach the baby, the baby is in observable somatic distress. The emotional power of these Bad Fits comes directly from the somatic passion that is aroused when the child–mother dyad is not satisfying. These somatic feelings are strong. They do not require words

DOI: 10.4324/9781032705835-5

for the baby to know they are there. They can be seen by the baby's facial or other body expressions. They become the springboard for the development of neuronal pathways that are formed in the right hemisphere. The Omnipotent Child develops as the container for the Bad Fits.

The Omnipotent Child is a construct to help therapists conceptualize and treat the origins of these highly resistant islands of identity that plague the patient and interfere with the development of a full, mature life. It is that part of the internal psychic structure that is the final common pathway of all passionately held Bad Fits that characterize not only the person's object ties and attachments but also his most powerful internal psychic identity. These early preverbal misattunements lay the early foundation for intimacy, identity, and conflict resolution.

Henry, a 40-year-old married man, entered therapy at the insistence of his wife to gain some insight into why his wife is always angry with him. During their courtship, the wife pursued Henry. Despite feeling he never really loved her, Henry married her. He was content being distant, but his wife, the pursuer, was not. He married the repeat of an early bad fit relationship with his mother. She was intrusive, and Henry, to protect his sense of self and the relationship, became passive. He tried to please his mother by being a good boy who was never angry, disruptive, or assertive. In describing his youth, Henry reported having difficulty sleeping, as well as feeling depressed, isolated, and not fitting in anywhere. In addition, he described having crushes on girls he could never call for a date. These feelings are Henry's Passionate Bad Fit. Henry learned that he constructed his Omnipotent Child to contain the Bad Fits in his life. He told himself, and lived by, "I am a loser and can't ever love anyone." This allowed him to keep reliving his early bad fits and not be abandoned. Henry was eventually able to see the futility of his Omnipotent Child. That led to Henry investigating steps toward living in a Passionate Good Fit.

The omnipotence referred to here is not the omnipotence of magical thinking or exaggerated views of oneself. It is the power of a fixed, somatically driven, island of identity. It feels as if it is indestructible, tenacious, and all-powerful over important aspects of the person's choices of attachments. It is particularly rigid around issues of mutuality and intimacy. The nature of the omnipotence demands to be highly idealized and held tightly with extreme loyalty. This loyalty can be heroic in maintaining, at all costs, the earliest Passionate Bad Fits. The child holds tightly to the unsatisfying early attachment in order to ward off a more chaotic and disorganized attachment. Through this, the child believes he saves his very own existence (Aledort, 2002).

The Passionate Bad Fit, contained in the Omnipotent Child, was described by me some time ago. Now, further research has clearly confirmed its power in the laying down of the neuronal pathways that regulate the right hemisphere systems. Schore (1991–2019) has shown that the central role of the right brain's unconscious mechanisms is to formulate and develop emotional communications and regulate affect in the early developmental stages. The right brain acts as a psycho-biological substrate of the human unconscious. It is in these areas that the Omnipotent Child resides and the bad fit flourishes. These early good and bad fits can have a dispro-portionate influence on the child's relationship to others, to his own body, and to his laying down of templates for intimacy and identity. When there are good fits, the child is able to be optimistic in his life, attach to a healthier person, be more curious of the world, take healthy risks, and feel as if his body was an ally, not an enemy who needs to be punished or denied.

Bad fits of early childhood leave the child with feelings of inadequacy, de-spair, fear of life, a profound distrust of his body, lack of curiosity with the world, and assumption of the worst in relationships. His identity is marked by a yearning for closeness that can become desperate but with very little knowledge of how to attach to another person (Aledort, 2002). These Good and Bad Fits are filled with strong somatic affect and excitement that tend to lay down the neu-ronal pathways in the right hemisphere. These passions imbue the child with an excitement that continually leads to the conscious and unconscious repetition of both these fits. These necessary re-enactments stabilize the early sense of self in the identity and in the body (Cohen, 2000). Such moments can lead to persistent, lifetime templates of unhealthy intimacy that people can, unfortunately, become quite heroic in maintaining.

The persistent existence of the Passionate Bad Fit serves to stabilize the early identity and create safety in a potentially harmful and stressful attachment. This is clearly the insecure attachment that needs to be stabilized, so it doesn't fall into a more chaotic and disorganized attachment (Stolorow & Lachman, 1980). It is not the repetition compulsion of Hendrick (1943) that was coined to explain the mastering of a difficult situation, where you can reclaim your self-esteem and not be humiliated.

How do we, as clinicians, see these insecure attachments being replayed, with heroic stature? How does the excitement get manifested and picked up by the thera-pist? The excitement, which is the very essence and sustainer of the bad fit intimacy, is usually hidden in the body or in the anticipatory phase of impending attachments and risk taking. The excitement can lead to body rashes, blushing, stammering, averting one's eyes, standing too close or too far away from someone, speaking in a way that cannot be understood or heard, by being too loud, by how one decides to dress, or by how one carries his body. It can lead to obesity or anorexia. There is also the anticipatory excitement of a bad fit. I don't know how many times I have heard patients complain of the intense anxiety that they have about coming home to a drunk husband, taking a test, going out on a date, going to work in the morn-ing, or trying to relate to a boss they hate or one who treats them terribly. These nervous anxieties are the very embodiments of the excitement of a Bad Fit and the Omnipotent Child in everyday life. All these forms of somatic excitement represent the expression of the bad fit intimacy that lives deep inside, with a need to sustain them. Contemplating losing them is terrifying. It is tantamount to a loss of identity.

What is striking initially in working with people who live in the hold of the Pas-sionate Bad Fit, or their Omnipotent Child, is their acknowledgment of how they cannot seem to control the situations they get into. They are aware of patterns in

their unsatisfactory relationships but feel helpless to change them and their behaviors. And, most of all, they have difficulty seeing their role in these relationships. They really have no knowledge of their Omnipotent Child. They have no
knowledge because the earliest formation of the Omnipotent Child is preverbal and
located in the somatic experiences of the first year of life. They cannot describe it
either verbally or visually.

I practice psychoanalytically oriented group psychotherapy in which the leader
has the central role. During the first phase of the group process, the leader is particularly crucial to the group. In subsequent phases, the leader assumes different
relationships to the group but always retains a crucial role in the group's work.
The leader is a transference object, a facilitator of group transferences, and makes
necessary interpretations to elicit the Passionate Bad Fits in the relationships in the
group. This is more akin to the relational–intersubjective approach (Stern, 2001),
where the therapist must enter the fray with the group to explore the Passionate Bad
Fits that are lying dormant. As the relationships are engaged, bad fits emerge. The
leader is quiet as the group does its work; he intervenes if the group stalls, becomes
defensive, or is resistant to the work.

From the outset, the work of the group is the fleshing out of the Omnipotent
Child. Exposing and working through the Omnipotent Child in the relationships
among group members, as well as in their own identities, invites the group members to contemplate change. The members struggle with giving up the Omnipotent
Child with its attendant emptiness and loss of identity. They struggle with taking in
a healthier identity, carrying with it new templates of intimacy and passion.

Like with the relational–intersubjective therapists (Stolorow, 2001), there is no
one theory that must be used. The theoretical models are secondary to the work of
fostering relationships in the group to explore the Omnipotent Child. Within these
parameters, the group leader uses the empathy and mirroring of self-psychology
(Segalla, 1996), the classical conflict theory of Freud, as well as the projective
identifications and the digesting of toxic introjects of Scharff (2001). All are used
to further explore the Omnipotent Child in group members. Empathy, introjects,
relationships, and conflicts dominate the themes. Preverbal experiences and the
search for words to describe them are highlighted. Particularly relevant are the
transitional, merged experiences, with their high-intensity affective moments. Underlying all the work is the developmental model particularly espoused by Mahler
(1968) and Pine (1985). In this model, the group goes through the same phases of
growth and development that a child goes through. In the beginning phase, there is
an inherent push for symbiosis, succeeded by pushes for separation–individuation.
These developmental phases are heavily influenced by the needs for excitement,
stimulation, curiosity, self-development, and the proclivity for bad and good fits
(Fonagy, 1999). These reflective functions can serve as either developmental
pushes or inhibitors.

When a patient calls seeking therapy, I set a time for our first meeting. Initial
sessions are an opportunity to both listen to what the presenting problems are and
to determine what type of therapy would be best for the patient. I do not take

psychotic or actively suicidal patients. Over time, I have found that many of my new patients have had previous therapy that has led to some changes in their life and in their feelings about themselves, but these changes have never felt substantial or permanent. I pay close attention to how the patient presents himself in story, affect, and somatic expressions. These can be important clues to his earliest preverbal difficult fits and the first step to help uncover the Omnipotent Child. Individual evaluation sessions are kept to a minimum so that potential transferences can occur in the group setting. I focus on those areas of the patient's life where he is particularly stuck. I ask about any particular physical feelings that coincide with the stuck position, such as headaches, stomach pain, neck or back pain, and locations of somatic anxiety. Further exploration of the patient's understanding of his stuck positions, including excitement, and good and bad fits is made. Every effort is made in these first sessions to introduce the concept of good and bad fits, the passionate attachments to them, and the Omnipotent Child.

I usually see patients twice for an evaluation. In the first session, they describe what hurts and for how long, their past history with any therapy, and whether they had specific feelings or dreams about their prior therapist. I tell them that they will most likely have some reactions to me or my office, and I encourage them to share those feelings with me. I highlight that this will be an important part of our work together. In addition, I take a family history, paying close attention to any evidence of early bad fits.

The second session usually begins with my asking if they have any thoughts, feelings, or questions about the first session. I also ask if they've had any dreams. We may then begin our mutual search for any known early bad fits in their life. I explain what the *passionately held bad fit* is and how that has made life difficult for most of my patients. I take a further history of their early life, their teen years, and the state of the family they grew up in. In particular, I ask about the family dinnertime and the feelings about that time in their lives. I comment, with empathy, about the difficult life they clearly had and how we are going to work on understanding it, how it happened, their role in it, and how we can change it. I point out any somatic expressions and ask what that means to them. I check on how they're managing the sessions so far. I explain that I will be important to them in our work, so it would be helpful if they could talk about any feelings they have toward me. I try to let them know that we will work together exploring and hopefully changing their basic concept of themselves. I might say, at this time, that they strike me as feeling that they could never love, that they are too angry, that they are doomed to always be a loser and never get the right guy or girl. I let them know that they have come by these ideas of themselves honestly and that they hold on to them too tightly and too heroically. I also let them know that we are going to do the work necessary to understand their early bad fits and how they still affect them. I usually recommend group as the best place to work out these issues I explain that it tends to take about four to five years and it is still more cost-effective than individual sessions. It is important that the patients know that there are responses that arise upon entering the group: fear, inability to articulate their story, anxiety about telling that story to strangers, feeling like they do not belong, and excitement. Then they begin to settle in with me as someone who is protective and understanding of their anxieties and who offers hope.

In this evaluation, I ask for dreams, especially recurrent dreams. The dreams highlight the patient's willingness to delve into and to appreciate the unconscious processes that we will be working with. Also, the dreams illuminate some early and present conflicts that will embody the Omnipotent Child. The way we talk about the dreams gives both of us clues as to how comfortable we can be with each other, as well as the level of resistance between us.

> An older patient in the first session recalled having a recurrent dream of practicing his profession with his father in multiple ways. He cried when describing his love for his father and how much he misses him. I asked him, "What about your mother?" He laughed and said, "I think it's why I'm here; because I do not treat my wife as well as I should."
>
> Another patient recalled recurrent dreams of bypassing his mother's house and going to his grandmother's house instead. This foreshadowed his struggle with assuming that any nurturing woman could not be where she should have been.

I try to be transparent in the evaluation by letting the patient know how hard this work will be, how the group process will most likely affect him or her, how we will most likely battle desperately against wanting to keep the Omnipotent Child, and my hope and struggle to help them move to a healthier place. I ask, "How are we doing? Do we like each other? Are we compatible with each other? What do you think of my office? We are going to spend a lot of time here together with 7 to 8 other people." It is important to keep checking in for a good or bad fit.

I let them know that I will be very present in the group process, and if either of us thinks at times that an individual session is needed we will have one. The group contract is explained. The group meets weekly for one and one-half hours. Confidentiality is required. There is no outside therapy. There is no involvement among group members outside the group room. In fact, group members do not know each other's last names.

Examples of Evaluation Sessions

Jack

Jack says he is unable to commit to anyone or anything, except for short periods of time. He is sad, but there is a smile of triumph as he explains the details of how he is difficult to capture. His smile belies the sadness in the situation. He says he was in love with a woman who ultimately left him for another man, and that is why he decided to try therapy again. Over the last six years, he had three failed therapy attempts. I point out that he seems to take great pride in his story of being the elusive one. He smiles again, goes on to excitedly tell more about his romantic life, and how he tends to regret many of his attachments. I let him know that he seems to be passionately involved in being elusive, and in living in regret. He seems to go from one bad fit to another, and I assume he will do the same in the group. Again, a big broad smile appears on his face. His Omnipotent Child is readily apparent.

> You will probably want to leave the group many different times, and hopefully you will learn something about your fear of intimacy that makes you want to run. Your fear of being captured by your mother has led your Omnipotent Child to be heroically able to escape any woman's wish to be close to you. I hope that we will be hearing more about where your father was. In this group, you may find your father as the one person in the group from whom you expect nothing. You will also have very mixed feelings about me, as I will be hard to make invisible.

I caught his attention, and he was no longer diffident, and instead looked puzzled and slightly irritated. "We will hopefully see this in the group. We have a lot of work to do and we should start now."

August

August is a 50-year-old man who is going through a divorce. He is cool, loose, glib, and, in his own way, seductive in the sessions. He describes a painful separation from his wife that is still unsettled. Both have hard feelings. He sees Iris, his current girlfriend, as the answer to all his problems. He then reveals, with a smile on his face, the multiple complaints Iris has about him. He clearly wants to satisfy Iris, just as he tried to satisfy his mother and wife. He is terribly blocked about his rage and disappointment with women. He tends to rephrase what I say without adding new information or insight into these dilemmas in his life. He is likable, but I am wary of his acting-out ability. In response to my questions about his passion, he says it is to be in love with Iris, go dancing, and be attractive to women. Previous therapy, designed to help him settle things with his wife, failed. He strikes me as a little boy who relies on magical thinking and a broad seductive smile and who hasn't the slightest idea of how to make a relationship work. I suggest to him that maybe his real passion is to be an adorable little boy who doesn't want to grow up. He doesn't resent the comment, which suggests to me that his need to be that little boy is a clue to his Omnipotent Child. I tell him he is going to be the cutest, most lovable little boy who won't grow up we have ever seen. "You will resist growing up, and the women in the group will try to love you, and I will try not to let them." He was both puzzled and slightly annoyed but with a whiff of relief. He then started the group and entered another crucial phase in his life cycle of his Omnipotent Child and Passionate Bad Fit.

Jane

Jane was referred by a friend from AA. She is an attractive woman in her 40s, with a big smile that belies her sadness, and has had many good and bad therapeutic experiences. As I was taking her history, she said that she was feeling surprised by some of my questions. For example, she said no other therapist ever asked her what she thought about them, or what she thought of their office. She was both pleased and puzzled by these questions. Again she commented, "In all of my work with other therapists, these questions about my feelings and fantasies about the therapist did not exist." She told me that recently she had trouble at her longstanding job. She thought it was because of a new, rather harsh boss, who thought that she made a mistake that he could not tolerate. She was angry and sad when telling this story. She had a difficult alcoholic father who, when displeased with her, would give her the silent treatment, something she found unbearable. She said her mother was ambivalent about her, and that five years ago her husband, whom she truly loved, died after a long illness. Her father died one year ago and she was in grief. She felt that she had gone beyond her grief. She was now with another man, who seemed, at times, to give her the silent treatment.

She was profoundly unhappy but tried her best to be upbeat. She said, "I'm not very nurturing or generous. I'm just like my mother." She told me that she heard from other patients of mine that I was tough. She felt I might be too harsh and not sympathetic enough, but she wanted to learn more. She was particularly interested in how we relate to each other since maybe, "I am acting out old stuff with my boss and with my boyfriend. I have missed that in my other treatments." I suggested that I would like to work with her in one of my weekly groups

In the second evaluation session, she was struck with how freeing it was for her to call me "harsh." It had not been easy for her to let people know when they have not treated her well. I commented that for most of her life, she lived in an unsafe family. Somehow, she found her good husband, and we needed to get her back to living in a Passionate Good Fit and help her live that way again. The group will do its best to help Jane do that. She was quite concerned about the safety in the group. She wondered, "What happens if someone wants to beat me up? Or someone dominates the room? Or no one wants to hear my sadness?" I tell her, "I try to be the lifeguard in the group and won't let people drown." She then revealed a more dangerous family situation with her father, which her mother clearly encouraged and allowed to develop. This situation existed for many years. She cried but with a smile. I told her that she seemed to keep trying to show me how she was not afraid, and how she could handle anything that was thrown at her.

I think this is your Omnipotent Child that you have lived in for most of your life. Right now, you are suffering from noticing that you cannot deal with all the losses, the job difficulty, and a new, difficult male friend, as easily as you thought you could. And your Omnipotent Child demands that you should be able to do all this heroically. Our job is to understand this Omnipotent Child, the Passionate Bad Fits you lived in, and, through the group and me, shift you to living in a Passionate Good Fit. I will try to notice when I am harsh, and do not expect you to live and endure that. Please call me on it if I lapse into harshness, and I will try to make sure that I figure out why I can come across as harsh to you.

Immediately she eagerly agreed to join the group. Afterward I thought: *Who in the group will take advantage of her adorableness? Who in the group will want to know her harshness? And who in the group will see her as making a mistake? I have to make sure that I do not give her the silent treatment, or, like her mother, let her get into difficult situations with some group members. I also need to figure out my "harshness."* These musings by me seem perfectly reasonable, but am I trying to make sure that the Bad Fits do not occur between us by trying to keep it too safe? Has she touched something in me that Jack and August have not? The work will continue for both of us.

Don

Don's initial contacts were unique. He was referred by one of my other patients. When he called to ask if I would see him, he immediately asked what the fee for the group sessions was. I told him; he got furious and scolded me: "You charge way too much. I would never pay that amount." Before I could respond, Don hung up. Six months later, he called again, asking the same question about the fee. I gave the same answer; he basically said the same things to me and hung up. I could tell how lonely he must be. Six months later, he called again. This time I said: "We both know the drill, but I really want to meet you and help you get through your rage at there being any fee for my services." He did not get mad; he listened and asked, "When can we meet?" One week later we met. I imagined him to be a gnarled, old, cantankerous, poorly dressed man, who was totally unlikable. He was some of that, but his history of child abuse, maternal neglect, and poor friendships made me think he needed lots of nurturing to comfortably be his 45-year-old, bright, highly educated, engineer self. Coming from Europe to live in the United States he had to adapt to a totally different culture. He sat uncomfortably in the chair that was the furthest away from where I sat. Where patients choose to sit can give clues about their difficulty finding the right distance between themselves and another person. It seemed Don still struggled to fit into the American culture. He told me that he never felt he belonged anywhere. He lived in his loneliness and anxiety. He felt reassured that I would do the right thing for him, since I knew his best friend. As the first session evolved, he seemed less anxious and a little more relaxed with me and with himself. He said he was afraid to start seeing me, since it felt like his last resort for a better life, and he didn't want to waste it. He said he came because his good friend told him he was foolish to not at least go for an evaluation. I suggested that perhaps he was repeating something from his history. I said, "It's no wonder you want to hold on to what you have, given your fear of this being your last resort." He looked puzzled by my comment, and I said that is the kind of work we will be trying to do here, hopefully in one of my groups. He was startled, then smiled and said that sounded courageous and exciting. We both smiled at that. I liked him and I felt he liked me.

Don began the second evaluation session by saying that he was able to pay the fee for treatment and that he liked my smile. I said, "Perhaps growing up you didn't have many smiles from your mother." I assumed that he had always longed for and needed a safe place to be. Unfortunately, he blamed himself for needing that safe place. He filled the rest of the session with many stories of how his mother neglected him, and how he tried to make her feel better. His efforts failed because his mother was in a constant battle with his out-of-control father. I pointed out that in our work in the group, he would have a chance to deal with his neglectful mother and terrifying father with the other group members. He asked why he should do that. I said,

> You need to do that, and I will be the lifeguard to make sure no one in the group drowns or gets hurt. You never had a lifeguard. You had to be your own lifeguard, and that task is impossible to do while simultaneously trying to live a happy mature life. In your effort to protect yourself you miss out on getting what you need. For example, your many early phone calls to me, which went on for a year, led to delaying getting what you needed. I'm glad you're here now so we won't further delay you working with me and me getting to know and understand you.

At this point, I felt that his Omnipotent Child was trying to be connected without having to take any risks. His Omnipotent Child kept him in a *status quo* position to allow him to live in the false hope that one day he'd have a better mother. He tearfully said, "I will lose all my hope for a better mother." I said that he will most likely repeat this important piece of his internal life in the group. I added that we would talk about hope in a different way—one that led to his being able to take risks in the group that can lead to fulfilling some of his hopes. He agreed to give it a try. I said I would need a one-year commitment so I knew that we would have time to work on these issues. He agreed.

Phases of Group Development

Phase One: The Symbiotic Mother

The task of this phase is to understand the earliest Passionate Bad Fits. During this early phase, when the group is chatting to get to know each other, I will usually interrupt and let them know that, for now, I am the most important person in the group. This comment usually leads to a great deal of consternation, anger, humor, and puzzlement. I use this technique to help the group fully appreciate the influence of the mother on the newborn baby. For example, in one group a woman began to fear that I would be unduly criticized by the group and wondered how she could protect and help me. I suggested that, as a young child, she had to protect and care for her mother instead of her mother caring for her. At the same time, there was a man who became furious that I would pretend to be his mother, and said that if I persisted he would either leave the group or make me leave the group. Both learned later how intensely traumatizing their childhoods had been, because of hating the mother, or having to rescue the mother from her distress.

In this phase, the group members are acutely sensitive to their own struggles and their intense feelings about me. A new member is left for me, consciously and unconsciously, to deal with. As the new member struggles with his early ambivalent fits, there is little empathy from others in the group. For example, a new member came into the group and asked if he could have one of the light bulbs dimmed, because it hurt his eyes. The group immediately told him he was wasting his time. The therapist would not change the bulbs. They told him to just stop asking and pay attention to the therapist. They were all too busy being infants with mother.

The therapist/symbiotic mother is always in the room. As this slow process of moving toward the mother in symbiosis unfolds, the struggle over the longing for the good fit collides with the exposure of the early misattunements. Many times the collision of desires, needs, and painful somatic introjects can lead to silence in a new member. It can also lead to excessive involvement with the other members, but, more often than not, it leads to a cascade of complaints about the physical environment of the group office.

The office in this phase of the work is the personification of the body of the infant–mother dyad. As such, it can become an expression of both contentment and discontent. When the group experiences a good-fit symbiosis with the mother, the room becomes a protective cocoon. This is evidenced by the inattention of the group to outside disturbances, such as the door being left open, knocks on the door, fire engines passing in the street, or the phone ringing.

When the group is caught up in describing their early bad fits, the room becomes a cacophony of discontent and irritation. Some complain about the temperature in the office, the shades being drawn incorrectly, or the noise out in the street. Many periodically complain about or admire the paintings in the office or the family photos. Others may express distress over the degree of stimulation in the group. Some feel it is too crowded, too quiet, too empty, or too dull. Some wish to bring food into the room, while others complain of there not being enough airtime. Such complaints are universal in group psychotherapy, but here they are processed differently.

These complaints set up the foundation for the inherent preverbal conflicts to emerge, and for the group to hold and contain the accompanying frustrations, anger, annoyance, and deep longings. Each new group member is gradually introduced to the concept of being in the therapist's lap. At no time is the fantasy acted out. This regressive fantasy construct helps organize and locate the earliest bad fits and the Omnipotent Child in the symbiotic relationship with the mother (who is the therapist). This fantasy construct also helps to organize and develop a group culture that allows, in successive phases, the further elucidation and fleshing out of the Omnipotent Child.

The fantasy construct of the therapist's lap is an integral component of the therapist assuming the role of the mother of symbiosis (Mahler, Pine, & Bergman, 1975). As the new member enters the ongoing group, the therapist continues his stance of the symbiotic mother. Simultaneously, the rest of the group struggles to know the internal life of the new member and his potential for relationships in the group. The new member invariably moves in the direction of the symbiotic mother with questions, incredulity, puzzlement, horror, shame, somatic feelings, suspicions, and highly ambivalent longings. The therapist, through his personal involvement and his attention to the new patient, encourages the regressive pull to the mother of symbiosis.

> Emily enters the group, and wraps herself in a hoodie, while trying to make her chair a lap for herself. She is a frightened little girl who complied with joining the group, but then, to her amazement, finds herself needing to hide. I let her know that she is letting us know, as all the new members had, about her earliest bad fits that were preverbal and resided in our bodies. I say, "You've told us a great deal of information that we'll develop together as we continue the work. How sad it must have been for you to feel there was no escape and you could only hide out." She struggles with her longings and fears of being seen at all. Her chief complaint is her inability to satisfy her professional goals. She was a failure all of her life. The group is able to empathize with her fears and need to hide, and wonders if she could imagine that the therapist's lap could feel safe.

I pull the interactions to myself, putting myself in the center of the action in the group. I actively comment on and ask questions about the new member's history and her reactions to the group experience. I may interrupt a dialogue that moves away from me, or even comment on how difficult it might be to "have me so big."

In this phase of the group process, the therapist deals with each of the complaints and feelings as examples of clues to early Passionate Bad Fits with the mother of symbiosis during the child's infancy. I assume these early complaints are the early misattunements around the mother–child dyad and their respective bodies in the feeding, touching, holding, and gazing phases (Beebe, 2000; Shore, 2002b). I posit that they are telling us the origins of the early nuclei for the formation of the Omnipotent Child, rather than fight–flight conflicts. As such, these early complaints are highly important. They are taken seriously and worked with in the context of their early relationships to the therapist and the group room. This differs from Rutan, Stone, and Shay (2007) and his developmental model.

In response to these complaints, the therapist says,

> I guess you're telling us how it wasn't right in those very early times with your body and your mother's body. You want it better, but you really don't expect it to be better in here. I'm sure you've experienced many things that just didn't fit right either in yourself, or in your relationships.

> In one session, Fran complains with great frustration that the room goes too fast for her. It gives her a headache; she feels unsteady, she gets confused. I respond to Fran, "How difficult it has been for you to regulate what is inside and what is outside of you. What would happen if you could permit yourself to imagine what it would be like to be in my lap? My lap is big enough to regulate what needs to be regulated." The typical responses to this invitation are incredulity, laughter, and confusion.

August jumped at the chance to be in my lap, and wanted to snuggle with me as long as he could. I told August that he knew that side of his relationship with his mother, but what about the part of him that didn't want to go near me and did not trust me. He looked puzzled and a little annoyed. Most ignore the lap, and the rest reject it at this time.

Jack, who has been in the group for three months, eloquently pleaded his case to resist the invitation. "My problem is with my father, not with my mother, and you are not my mother. I've already idealized you as my father. So far you haven't done anything wrong to me or to anyone else in the group. My mother is the bitch and she needed me to idealize her. I'm too angry to be too close to her and you can't be her." I reply, "What happens if I'm talking about you as an infant and me as your mother trying to redo what went wrong in those early years?" Three sessions later he responds by saying, "I don't know if you can take my feelings toward my mother. I've been in therapy before. I know all the answers, and why should you be able to help me? I could do it myself." I respond, "We've started our dialogue already. You're telling me how, as an infant, you must have felt in your body that your mother needed you to make her feel great, rather than the other way around. You knew, before words, that you had to do it on your own and you're not sure, nor should you be, whether I could suspend my own need for idealization and gratification, and pay enough attention to you." That idea interests him and he asks for more information about this construct. He receives a great deal of support for this attempt to be in my lap.

Fran admits, with a great smile, how she already is in my lap, but in a different way. She fantasizes that I am a large sheepdog, who she can snuggle up to and feel safe with. She then laughs with the group about how this dog still has to be a work dog, and be responsible for all the sheep.

Through these intense, passionate, exciting interactions around the therapist's lap, I ask them to remember whatever they can about these early bad fits in their life. I ask for family myths about their infancy, and I let them know that they most likely felt this way in all their important passionate relationships.

Jane tries to become a good group member by not making any demands on the group, yet she notices whenever she feels that I have been "harsh" to her or others in the group. She says that she was very "harsh" when she was younger to men in her life. Her father was mean to her mother and then she would retaliate against him by giving him the silent treatment. I say, "Do you think you give me the silent treatment, by only focusing on my harshness? You try your best not to address me. Seeing me as harsh seems to protect you and the group from having to take care of your mother and fight her battles. You smile a great deal, and that strikes me as an adorable little girl who would like me to protect her from the rest of the group. Instead, you're trying to protect them from me as the harsh parent. Your complaint is that you cannot find a good man for yourself. Maybe if you tried to notice the feelings inside of you when you see me as not harsh, a new and different fit may evolve. You could get closer to finding the proper man for yourself." The older group members, who have been through this, laughingly tell Jane that "he is just trying to have you fantasize about getting into his lap." A borderline woman in the group, who has been chronically depressed, cries and reports to the group that if she got into my lap, her whole life of despair, agony, pain, and revenge on her parents, and her miserable childhood, would be for naught. Her whole *raison d'etre* would be for nothing. One man says, "His lap was offered to me when I came in, and I've refused it for about a year, because if I got into his lap I would pound his chest until he bled. I would kill him off and then where would I be? I still need a good mother, I guess. He tells me that he can tolerate it, but I don't believe him." Another patient tells the new member that if she got into my lap, she would be concerned that I would get aroused, as her sexually promiscuous father did. Another man proudly announces that he still hasn't taken my offer. Now he wonders that maybe he is mistaken. Another says that he still wants to be mad at his mother, no matter what the cost is to him and the group.

The older members now aid in eliciting the earliest passionate bad fits in the patient's life as well as his potential for the bad fits in the group. They aid in the development of the regressive pulls by exploring with each other their own history of bad fits and how they expect the new member to have them as well.

The Omnipotent Child is fleshed out in this phase through the intense, somatic, passionate, mutual experiences among the therapist as the mother of symbiosis, the new member, and the rest of the group. There is lots of giggling, anger, despair, and helplessness in reliving and discussing these early bad fits. There is a great deal of suspicion and mistrust at any hint of a good fit in the group, which gives further evidence of the power of the Omnipotent Child. The Omnipotent Child construct is re-introduced, and the group begins to try to understand the nuances of the powerful effects it has in their lives.

The following case examples are from the same twice-weekly group that has met over the last five years. They demonstrate, in more detail, the interactions between the group and the therapist that elucidate the Omnipotent Child in various phases of their development in the group and in their lives.

Phase One: August

August comes into the room as if he has been there all his life. He shows little anxiety that might be expected in a new situation. He proceeds to tell his story without much encouragement. He is a tall, attractive man whom the women and men quickly notice. He fills his end of the sofa, spreading out in a non-August manner. He describes his marriage as unfixable. Since his separation, he has been dating Iris. His self-involvement is immediately evident and, except for his wish that I help him with Iris, he complains of nothing. At first, the group is tolerant of his self-centeredness and preachy manner, but as the irritability heats up, Frank speaks to the group's outrage at August's indifference and smugness as he tells him, "You better get into the therapist's lap now and learn something different about yourself, before you get hurt. The therapist's lap is big enough for all of us." August replies that his father was useless and I would most likely be just as useless. August has contempt for the invitation. He continues to refuse the lap. He gets into more and more trouble in the group with his alternating condescension and obsequious manner. He treats the group the way he and his mother treated his father.

To both protect him from being scapegoated and to get him into the symbiotic mother's lap, I make several interpretations over time such as,

> As long as you avoid me and my lap, and your early experiences with your mother, the more you're going to treat the group as the degraded father. This recreates for you your special passionate attachment to your mother at the expense of your father and your own adult manhood. It's costing you a lot to protect that early, special, passionate relationship with your mother. It seems that your early passionate bad fit with your mother was your sense, in your body and in hers, that you were the most incredible little boy she had ever seen, and neither of you needed anyone else, especially not your father. You're caught up with your girlfriend in an erotic, aggressive cocoon that we must all look at but not touch.

I tend to make comments that are a mixture of interpretation and explanation, are body-oriented and immediately present. His confusion and indignation are the first signs of his passion in the group. This encourages me. I both protect and put demands on him through my invitation, persistent gaze, and focus. My comments come from the need to have him know a respected and powerful father in this group.

Over time, August reveals his story with his mother. He was the overly adored child conceived in an affair mother had that was kept secret until his mother died. He lives with deceit, secrets, and enduring shame. His Omnipotent Child is his being overvalued by his shameful mother and, as such, he needs to stay oblivious to reality, as his mother had. "I will be loved no matter what I do," he says. "I can't understand how people don't like me. I can't understand why I am hurt so easily when my wife, and now my girlfriend, snub me, and question my love for them." I tell him many times, in many different ways, that the most passionate moments in his life (his Omnipotent Child) are being adored insincerely by his shameful mother. I explain how he eagerly looks forward to living in this bad fit because when he is in this bad fit he knows his identity in a clear way. His intimacy experiences have to be marked by insincere adoration by both partners. Attempts to relive it are made by his excessive loving or "breakfast in bed," as he was served throughout his adolescence.

He found sitting in my lap protective, sad, and, much to his amazement, soothing, but not overstimulating as he had feared. The exposure of his Omnipotent Child gave the group a chance to be empathetic to him. He is able to see, for the first time, his old relationships, his new one with his girlfriend, and his being provocative in the group. He is now struck with how he can see his behavior through a different lens.

Phase One: Don

Don's first contact with me is to schedule an appointment for an evaluation. He ends each call angrily. He is either angry over the fee or the available times we can meet. After three months, we finally agreed on an appointment time. Shortly thereafter, Don enters the group process, with reluctance, suspicion, and resentment. He tells me that he desperately needs to fix his relationships with women. He can't imagine it is possible to do this, especially not in a setting with women.

In Don's first phase of the group, he is continuously angry, irritable, and obnoxious to the women. He complains about most things in the group room. I comment to Don many times that he won't let anyone, especially me, hold him and be a source of comfort for him. He keeps trying the women in the group but turns them off, and they see him as an incorrigible and needy pest. He acts like a child with eczema or colic who can't be quieted down or lulled to rest. He did have colic as a child, he sadly and reluctantly reports. At times he stammers. At other times he will unconsciously rotate his arms as if he is a rooster ready to crow. He is shocked that these movements are noticed by the group. He was always ashamed of them and never could understand why they were part of his body. At this time, he is content to know that they were part of his very painful preverbal life with colic and a mother who was so frustrated at not being able to comfort her child. Just knowing that there could be an explanation for these bodily movements led to the beginning of trust and hope to have his preverbal experiences understood by me and the group. I comment that his early relationships, particularly the preverbal ones, most likely were filled with tension, ambiguity, and distrust. He becomes sad, cries, and tells us that is what he imagines as well. His mother never gave him anything without extracting a price. His Omnipotent Child keeps him in a passionate, angry, maddeningly distrustful state of longing for his unavailable mother, and women like his wife.

The women in the group can now have empathy for Don's treatment of them. They continually point out to him how he sets himself up to be rejected so he can make his Omnipotent Child real, and live in the Passionate Bad Fit. He feels stuck now. What could he do with women who want to hold and comfort him, in a lap that soothes him, lets him rest, and satisfies his ancient longing? When Don withdraws and becomes silent and even sometimes naps, I let Don know the importance of his being able to take rest periods from the demands of the symbiotic mother. He struggles mightily with his conundrum in the group, and in himself. Can he surrender the Omnipotent Child for something better, or is he going to remain loyal to it, and its splendid passionate isolation?

During this intense struggle, in which the whole group is able to identify with and recount their own Omnipotent Child, and their own loyalties, I stress to Don and the group how powerful these loyalties are. I say,

The Omnipotent Child defines not only your template of intimacy in relationships, but also your very early identity. To give up the Omnipotent Child at this phase in your work, you will have to trust the group to hold you and be there as you live in the unknown until you find a newer identity, based on good fits. The group is the best place and structure to hold someone in the terrifying unknown for as long as they need to be held, understood, and not taken advantage of during their vulnerability.

The multiple identities in the group help to cushion the change and to allow a newer identity to form (Frederickson, 2000). In this phase of the group, which can last about one and a half years, the constructs of the therapist's lap, the symbiotic therapist, and the persistent working with the preverbal influences on identity, intimacy, and conflict resolution set the stage for the deepening of the work into the separation–individuation phase of development, and further struggles with the need to hold on to the Omnipotent Child at all costs.

Phase Two: Separation and Individuation

Frank engages the fantasy of the lap for about a year. During this time, he is able to complete the separation from his wife. He lets the women in the group find him appealing and tender. He comments that this is the first time in his life that he believes that a woman could find him attractive and lovable. He needs to try on his new identity in the group and leave the lap. Almost immediately, he gets himself into trouble in the group. His new-found identity fills him with a new sense of power. He doesn't know how to use it, or what to do with it. He is now seen as loud, arrogant, and intolerant of others' pain. He finds himself alone and scared in the group. I beckon him back into my lap until he can negotiate his separation and individuation from the good-enough mother. He needs intermittent refueling stops in the therapist's lap. In a short course of time, he is able himself to ask to come back and forth into the lap until he gets it right. This process leads to the unveiling of another potent Omnipotent Child that occurred at the time of separation–individuation. He begins to be angry with me, this time in his nightly dreams. He sees me as his jailer, and he is my prisoner. I won't let him have fun with the women in the group, or in his outside life. I won't understand how much he hurts. I won't let him go. I hold on to him too tightly. I don't like his newfound swagger and power. I need him to be in my lap and not the other way. He brings in these nightly fights with me. As he reports these dream fights, he begins to smile and clearly enjoys them. The fights allow him the right distance to be close to mother and to me. I, too, look forward to his dreams, as I find them fascinating. I let him know that I enjoy his newfound power, which is to engage me in an exciting relationship that appears safe to both of us. The group admires his power, which allows his arrogance to be modified and transformed. I reaffirm for him his desire to be close, to be one with me. I also confirm for him his intense fear of being held captive in that longing state without escape. We all help Frank define his Omnipotent Child in this phase of his development in the group.

Frank tries to speak about his earliest years, which he can remember only in his body. He talks hesitantly, reminding all of us of his stuttering as a child, and how big-bosomed his mother was. He assumes he was held tightly by his mother in her large breasts, since she tended to do that when he was older. He remembers her perfume and feels silly and ashamed of that recollection. He assumes that his mother held on to him so that he couldn't move away from her. He feels he must have been rocked often, as he loves to rock today. As we work through this preverbal period, his tears are always mixed with anger and the feeling of being imprisoned. I speculate with him that the imprisonment might be due to his being held too tightly by his mother, and how helpless and angry his body felt to be stimulated by the excessive holding and squeezing. The intimacy with his mother in his earliest years may have felt by his body as if it was too much, too tight, too intense, and too inconsistent. He pays a high price to be stuck in his Omnipotent Child. I need to be sure I don't hold on to him too tightly. I need to create a dialogue with him so we can explore this together with the group. His Omnipotent Child, in this phase, is how passionately and heroically he can stay in jail.

Phase Three: Sexuality, Ambiguity, and Safe Harbors

While the group works with August and Frank, Brenda is not a silent participant. Brenda always sees herself as a loser, damaged goods, a victim, asexual, and barely better off than her alcoholic parents. She is basically sad, depressed, and over-whelmed with life and its demands. Previously, Brenda had individual treatment that she felt helped a little, but never got to her "core." Brenda can also be charming and good-humored. The group takes to her immediately as the group's "mascot." She is both flattered and confused by this designation. She is the embodiment of the failed, inadequate life, and the projection of the group's own sadness and child-like bad fit yearnings. She represents the sexual inadequacies in the group, as well as the emptiness in their relationships and in themselves. Her Omnipotent Child is defined and exposed as that part of her that passionately lives in the identity of the failed and inadequate woman. It is hard for Brenda to hear that she longs for the next failure in her life, and celebrates it as best she can. She brings in weekly stories of her inadequacies and failures in negotiating life in general. I use her mascot position as the group's need to celebrate her failures and not notice the cost and the harm to her. When the group takes back their own projections onto Brenda, they begin to appreciate the power of her Passionate Bad Fit, and how she holds on to it as the only close relationship she ever had. While sitting in the fantasy of the therapist's lap, new and different demands are made on her. Her victim storytelling is interpreted as her attempt to seduce the group and hide her power from herself and the group. The therapist holds her in a demanding, powerful lap that refuses to accept her sad stories. Her Omnipotent Child is defined as how she is going to be the most passionate victim in the group with the saddest stories.

As Brenda begins to individuate from the lap and her Omnipotent Child, she comes under the protection of a powerful, highly effective woman in the group.

This woman protects Brenda, cajoling her to notice the group and how they work in a different way. Now my demands are that she notices the other women and men in the group. I ask that she talk about what she notices about the other people and how they manage their lives. She periodically comes in with another sad story. To this I respond, "I'm not your failed mother who needs you to be like me. I expect you to be tougher, and I won't abandon you if you are." I know that Brenda is on her way to individuation when she reports a dream in which she invents a "coring machine" and "cored me out," laughing all the way.

Brenda's separation–individuation phase is highlighted by many trips back and forth to my lap and the group's lap. Eventually, she begins to present herself more as a sexual being. She begins to wear different clothes, changes her hairstyle, and gets a personal shopper under the direction of the women in the group. She is still the group's mascot but in a healthy way. She blossoms and leads the way to the next phase of development in the group, which includes issues of sexuality, ambiguity, and safe harbors.

As Brenda matures in the group and starts to feel like a woman, she falls in love with Mel. Mel, still struggling from a childhood fusion with a psychotic, seductive mother, becomes the man in Brenda's life. How are the group and Brenda going to talk about her sexuality and the ever-present sexuality in the group? The task of this phase is for the group to create a safe harbor from the regressive pull toward the fantasized, retaliatory, pre-oedipal, phallic mother, or "witch mother," who experiences these newer feelings as disloyalty to her. The group must allow the father to come in as the protective parent in order for the process to continue. The group must now deal with the discovery of the sexual differences among the members, and their concomitant anxieties, gender confusions, fantasies, and primal scene recollections. They must also contend with their Omnipotent Child and its need to recreate the Passionate Bad Fit with other members in the group around these issues. In this phase, Brenda actively struggles with her internal need to go back and be the depressed, inadequate mother who rejects the new, arousing feelings of excitement in her body, and in her fantasies. She could serve an important function for the group to be that depressed, rejecting mother. The therapist focuses on this dynamic to move the group to the next phase but also to expose further the Omnipotent Child that resides in this developmental phase. I say,

It must be hard to imagine that the passion of making love to Mel could ever match the exquisite passion of being the asexual, overwhelmed little girl in the arms of your inadequate and depressed mother. What choice are you going to make? We'll hold you while you decide to leave your Omnipotent Child and join us in the fray in here with the group and tolerate being excited. Someone else most likely will take your role as the depressed mother.

I now actively engage in facilitating dreams, sexual fantasies, and group member attachments. At the same time, I ensure a safe harbor from the enraged, abandoned, and pre-oedipal parent. This safe harbor is structurally reinforced by the firm boundaries that are set in the group from the outset. When regressive fantasies occupy the group, they feel real, and the boundary between fantasy and reality is always attended to. I am constantly looking for the group's ambivalent relationship to the excitement and arousal toward each other and in their bodies. In the context of this phase, I encourage Mel and Brenda to verbally explore their feelings of excitement and anxiety toward each other, as well as toward their bodies. Both their Omnipotent Children come roaring out in this context. Mel declares, in many ways, that he can only get close to women who are going to make him feel crazy and absorb him. Brenda represents a safe harbor for him. She is a female with whom he can lead the way, where he can feel in charge. Mel spends most of his life either in three difficult marriages or in isolation to protect him from women. Brenda helps Mel move from his position of isolation, to try again with a different woman. He is more able to do this, now that he has a protective father and a safe harbor in the group. Brenda now captivates the group by her intense sexual fantasies with Mel. She exclaims that this passion, in fact, is better than being the victim with her mother. She is now seen as a worthy competitor, which provokes a great deal of anxiety in her, and a longing to return to her Omnipotent Child. She vacillates on that cliff of the unknown for months, before she decides to let herself be seduced by someone other than her depressed mother. Mel is anxiously forthright and direct with Brenda in talking of his warm, loving, sexy feelings toward her.

In this phase, I alternate being the mother of symbiosis, who can still and always be present for the patients who need to return for protection, to catch their breath, to feel safe, and to continue growing, with allowing myself to be a more obvious transference object, and therefore having to deal with my own narcissistic injury of not being the most important person in the group room.

Phase Four: The Analytic Culture

This last phase of the group's development is the culmination of the previous stages. It becomes the analytic culture that sustains the group forever. It is here that the Omnipotent Child finally gives way, to be replaced by a more mature understanding and empathy for the origins of the Omnipotent Child and the intense need to hold on to it. The power of the Omnipotent Child is lessened. Patients are freer to pursue different and better fits. They can better tolerate the concomitant anxiety of their shifting to newer identities. Now patients are more able to recognize the regressive shifts. August can now appreciate the experience of being taken seriously and respected by the group, rather than being the adored man/child of mother and the world. Frank now notices that he puts himself in jail with his new woman and knows what it is about. This phase tolerates and invites the sadness, rage, and depression of giving up the old Passionate Bad Fits and loyalties.

Mel makes progress in understanding his Omnipotent Child. However, he remains reluctant to join the therapist in the fantasy of the lap, seeing it as much too dangerous and exciting. Under the influence of Brenda's sexual overtures, and his concomitant arousal, Mel regresses to a "safer" homosexual position with Bob, which backfires. Mel talks in a soft, seductive voice, which is labeled by Bob as his "pied piper" voice. Mel attempts to lure Bob to be close to him in a way that feels unhealthy because of the hidden aggression. Bob rails against Mel and his seductive manner, as it stirs up homosexual anxiety in him and the group. Mel is very close to being scapegoated and thrown out because of the anxieties he stirs up in the men. This fits perfectly with his earlier Passionate Bad Fit relationships with both father and mother, which were highly eroticized and laden with aggression. Mel lets the group know how both his parents seduced him. At this point, I again invite Mel into my lap for his protection as well as a place for him to appreciate his highly eroticized aggression and passionate attachment to it. The fantasy experience of having Mel in my lap is quite extraordinary. I feel as if he disappears inside of me. Mel validates that. He says that he doesn't just sit in my lap but, in fact, goes inside my heart and into my blood system. He wants to feel the warmth of my blood and to know me in a way that he never knew anyone else. He asks if he can stay for as long as he wants; I agree. It doesn't feel as if I am invaded. It feels like a warm, loving fusion that doesn't arouse homosexual feelings. He needs someplace to be inside without the aggression. During this time, he becomes rather silent in the group, avoiding provocative invitations from Bob. He feels an internal quiet. As Mel is in my lap, which doesn't occur until he is in the group for about two years, the discussion around it quiets the homosexual anxiety in the room and makes it possible for the group itself to discuss and examine their homosexual longings. Mel begins to understand how his Omnipotent Child was the passionate attachment to the quandary of either being alone and stuck in the longing for someone to be close to, or disappearing inside someone. As he works through his rage and sadness about his mother, and how confusing and anxiety-producing this relationship is, he becomes more available to the people in the room and to himself. He begins to notice, without anxiety this time, Brenda's struggle with her femininity and sexuality, and is drawn into her concerns. How could he be close to Brenda and still keep his newfound father, in the body of the group and the therapist? Brenda and Mel both need fathers to help separate them from their earliest attachments to their mothers and their bad fits. Their anxiety of inviting each other inside is defused by the earlier experience of Mel being inside of me. I use the bridging techniques of Ormont (1992) to facilitate their involvement with each other. Mel's Omnipotent Child is continually examined as he tries to move to a newer identity and form a relationship with Brenda.

During this time, Mel threatens to leave the group. He complains bitterly of losing his freedom, of not being in charge of his life anymore, of wanting to help Brenda but not wanting to be responsible for her. He feels trapped by the group and wants to run away. Most of all, he feels powerless to recapture his old Omnipotent Child, and rails against me for robbing him of it. He feels that people are getting too close to him. Brenda tells him that he sounds like she did when she got here. She implores him to imagine with her that their passion would be better than their old Omnipotent Children. In this context, he reports a series of dreams of redoing his mother's house and his own house. The group reminds him that the anxiety he feels is a result of seeking a newer identity with Brenda at this time. Over a period of four months, he moves among despair, anger, and rage toward himself, the group, me, and the exciting feelings of closeness with Brenda. I repeatedly comment that his Omnipotent Child is loosening its ties to him, and he doesn't really know how to feel or know who he is. His old bad fit identity is at stake now. The group reassures Mel, as they are intimately involved in this whole process of letting go of their own Omnipotent Child for something better with someone in the group. Mel begins to feel the impotent rage of his wasted years living with his Omnipotent Child. His despair turns to sadness and abject misery. While this is going on with Mel, Brenda reports dreams of how she has a deformed baby attached to her arm that she is to carry for the rest of her life. She assumes that the deformed baby is her Omnipotent Child. Months later, she reports another dream of how the baby is now separated from her body. She is now on a train traveling to unknown places. When she sees the parents of this baby, she gives the baby back to them. Mel then complements her dreams with his dream of being locked up in a boat with a ferocious bear that he decides he can handcuff by himself, which he very proudly does. He experiences the dreams that he shares with Brenda as their union together as well as his moving to another and newer place in his life and inside of him. The bear is his Omnipotent Child. He recognizes that it isn't as ferocious as he thought. He can handcuff the bear. (In the group I sometimes think of myself as a mother bear protecting her cubs.) Both Mel and Brenda celebrate their new relationship to their respective Omnipotent Children, and to their new relationships with themselves. Mel and Brenda get closer. Brenda learns to masturbate for the first time and to feel loved. Mel is able to be close to a woman without feeling swallowed up. The group acknowledges that their dreams are a love song between them of new identities, with new passions and, more importantly, new found templates of intimacy.

The intense anxiety and helplessness that Mel feels as he gives up living in his Omnipotent Child is profound for him and the group. Mel and Brenda's sexually charged union stirs the group members to look at their own Omnipotent Child in the realm of excitement and arousal. One year later, Mel leaves the group, after being there for four years. He feels closer to his daughter than ever before, more open about his competitiveness, and more comfortable living by himself. Brenda keeps smiling. A number of years after Mel leaves the group, Brenda gets married.

The Omnipotent Child may be present in all phases of a child's development and therefore will be present in all phases of the group work. The Omnipotent Child reveals itself rather quickly in the evaluation sessions and continues to do so in the group work. The therapist repeatedly identifies the Omnipotent Child for the patient and other group members. Through the continued interactions among the group members and the therapist, be they active or silent, the repetitive, stuck positions are identified and examined in detail. Focus is directed at the intense holding onto positions taken in the group and with themselves or with the therapist. Any position, be it complaining, depressive, shaming, enraging, grieving, whining, provocative, seductive, infantile, or avoidant, comes under Omnipotent Child scrutiny. The somatic component is inquired about. Over time, the power of the early preverbal experiences is introduced. The group is asked to struggle with trying to understand this power, to make it conscious and alive, to put it into words, not to leave it buried only in their bodies. The notion that they are holding on to their positions as a way to re-experience the passion that they felt at an earlier time in their bodies and in their lives is introduced. Kernberg (2001) discusses the impact of high-intensity and low-intensity affect on the earliest formation of unconscious fantasies and their organizing structures. Schore (2002b) also emphasizes the role of early affect intensity in the formation of the self. This is closely akin to the role of passion in the development of the Omnipotent Child. The idea that the Omnipotent Child enables the member to stabilize and solidify his earliest identity (Cohen, 2000) at any cost is also examined in the group. The resistance to these demands is worked with as aspects of their Omnipotent Child as well.

Through identifying and working through the Omnipotent Child in group psychotherapy, patients are able to move to a new and firmer identity with a different, healthier, and more mature template of intimacy. It is important that the group focus on all the variations of the Omnipotent Child as it changes during all the developmental phases. The therapist and the group must comment on the attendant anxieties as the Omnipotent Child demands more and more loyalty and heroism to sustain it as the only intimate, profound attachment in their lives. The group focuses on the anxiety as being related to the shifting of identities and the concern of not knowing who you are. There is enormous relief in understanding the anxiety and despair in this manner. The patients, and the group, use it to continue the work in seeing the anxiety as a sign of positive change. These examples show the movement within a group of how the Omnipotent Child is manifested, how the therapist helps to expose the Omnipotent Child, and how the analytic culture, which is developed over time, ultimately helps with working through the Omnipotent Children of different phases. This focus on the Omnipotent Child is particularly gratifying to patients who have been in previous treatments but have never really changed their internal structure.

Part 2

Shame

Shame is a subject that has been overlooked and neglected. This section examines shame from a distinctive new perspective when working with the human condition. This brings out the need for the therapist to always be aware of the hidden shame and act accordingly.

DOI: 10.4324/9781032705835-6

Chapter 5

Concepts of Shame and the Excitement in Shame

Shame is omnipresent and tends to be hidden, even though it is one of the most powerful affects in our emotional system. It comes from failures in relationship to the internal ego ideal, and the regressive desires of longing for others. Alonso & Rutan, 1988 believe that shame is a primary affect arising from the earliest autistic position, and it therefore lives in an isolated, autistic state that keeps itself hidden, as if in a cocoon. This corresponds to the earliest preverbal relationship and the nucleus of the Omnipotent Child experiences.

The earliest origins of shame can be seen in the infant–mother dyad. If the dyad doesn't allow sufficient holding and good-enough fits, then the Passionate Bad Fits arise and include shame as the leading affect to express this dilemma. At the same time, if the dyad doesn't allow independence and grandiosity of the self to be explored and experienced, shame will be the exciting affect that will stabilize these bad fit or Omnipotent Child identities in their body ego, hence their ego ideal, and then their sense of self as the dyad and the individual develops. These internalized self-states then influence the intimacy that the individual will move toward as a way to stabilize these Passionate Bad Fit relationships. Group therapy experience heightens both these positions. The group raises self-consciousness and the regressive longings for the other. These constructs are in constant tension.

Clinically, there are many ways that shame can present itself in the patient and in the group as a whole. One of the most common ways is with patients who come in with a history of failing at things, of not being able to attain the success they want to, and who are always in trouble with their bosses. They might be feeling shame about the fact that they're not the man they want to be, the husband or family man. They often present as feeling like they are an imposter, always waiting to be found out, or feeling episodes of anxiety and depression around their performance. This shame can certainly fit into the failure of the patient living up to his or her ego ideal. Another form is a shame that comes from post-traumatic experiences, either in the body or elsewhere. The post-traumatic shame can present as a tendency to blame themselves for dilemmas that they believe put them in the situation that led them to a traumatic event and to blame themselves intensely for not recovering soon enough or not succeeding in the face of the trauma.

DOI: 10.4324/9781032705835-7

One kind of shame, *somatic shame*, occurs when the body is invaded and abused; examples of this are anorexia or bulimia, obesity, people who have been attacked or raped, and people who have been traumatized early in life as infants. Another form of shame goes back to early preverbal forms of experience with failure, and this shame, I believe, is inexorably linked to identity and intimacy in the patient's life, without any real hope of getting past it. Another form of shame is the *heroic shame* that some people can wear as a form of identity; they are able to smile and lead a damaged life around them, and at the same time feel incredibly shameful about who they are and what they do.

The missing piece that keeps the shame hidden is the excitement and passion in the shameful experiences. I will present case examples of groups that struggle with these issues. The therapist's role is to find and search for the hidden excitement in the shameful positions. Gans, 2018 talks about defenses against shame in the group, like the group focusing on similar issues like loss or failure that are safe and avoid envy, competition, and longings. He also mentions disdain, guilt, and group collusive behavior, like all coming late without comment. Self-righteous indignation is another hallmark of the Passionate Bad Fit and its hidden shame and excitement. Shame cannot be worked through, unless you have worked through the hidden excitement and passion in the shameful moments or identities. Shame must be brought forth and put into relationships in the group, even though it can lead to further regressions, but it is also the only chance to work through and redo the earliest vulnerabilities. The earliest preverbal experiences that people suffer are usually dealt with by primitive defenses such as denial, repression, projection, and somatic excitement. It is this somatic excitement that is as powerful as the other defenses and is an integral part of the experience of shame and the disintegrative anxiety in the early preverbal experience. When the body ego is threatened, the earliest sense of self is threatened as well.

The space of shame usually gets replaced by an emptiness that is quite profound, as it recalls the passionate and hateful longings and hatred of themselves for their failures. There is also a profound regret at the decisions that were made, with the Passionate Bad Fits as the driver behind them. There is always the longing to return to the original states of shame, to solidify identity, and to decrease the anxiety of the beginnings of a new Passionate Good Fit.

Case Examples

Mary

The shame connected with Mary's conflict is being seen as grandiose and narcissistic vs. her attempt to resolve it by marrying narcissistic men and staying connected with them. She needs to cover up and hide her powerful wish to be in the limelight, even though she knows that she has the tools to be there. Her shame is connected to her mother's desire to wipe out Mary's greatness, so her mother could be the only great woman in the house and community. A good example occurs when Mary does something outstanding—she sometimes will fall and trip, which humiliates her and brings her back to her powerful and organizing Passionate Bad Fit of shame. I asked her what was more exciting for her: doing well in the course, or waiting for and expecting to trip and fall and humiliate herself? The group talked a great deal about her excitement in anticipating the worst: the trip, the fallen position, and the anxiety. I would sometimes add, "Thank God for the falls. Who would we be if not for the anticipated and excited states of waiting for the falls?"

As she has begun to see her passion in the fallen position, she has begun to take steps in the direction of her own power and has begun to separate from the narcissistic men in her life. She is more connected to a man in the room, George, mired in his shameful Omnipotent Child about the profound loss of his innocence at too early an age, and not being able to rescue himself or his mother or sister from his toxic father. She is the bright star in his world in group. She now has to deal with her own wishes to be outstanding, out front, and, in my language, big and full of exciting fantasies of her future, her body, and her life. She can desire and find a man, while being the big one. She has been able now to stand out in the group, as she takes on a co-therapist role. She has let herself stand out by coming late to a few sessions and tolerating both the critical and the admiring gaze of the group. With great prompting, she was finally able one day to sing to the group—she is studying opera right now—and was warmly appreciated through the applause and the tears in the group.

The group discussed at length how each one of them would make themselves feel shameful. One would become overwhelmingly anxious about not passing a test, even though she knew the work exceptionally well, and was worried about being envied. Martin would wrap himself in his shameful intense sexual fantasies throughout the day, where these fantasies really expressed merging with the woman. This was a way for him to not appreciate the shameful neediness that he felt about wanting to merge with his mother and with his wife, which he warded off. The excitement in the sexual fantasies was a way not to notice, but to keep alive, shameful feelings that he was not the proper man he wanted to be. He couldn't let himself be the grandiose little boy he wanted to be because that meant killing off of his brother, as well as his passive father. This reenactment was beautifully crafted by him. When Myrna, who had the ability to weaken me and to make me more passive, was doing her thing, Harry did his. He acknowledged later on that when Myrna was "weakening" me, he began to elaborate some very intense sexual fantasies about her. The group helped him link together his history of sexual fantasies about his aunt, who was a very attractive woman, and his passive father.

Mary has struggled mightily for most of her life to thwart her romantic feelings and sexual fantasies for her highly narcissistic father, who was seductive, an alcoholic and an adulterer, and a powerful object in her life. Her attempts to hide her shameful feelings led her to gain 200 pounds in adolescence and to hurt her body for its insistence on having these shameful feelings and fantasies. This is a good example of the body as enemy, not ally. Not only did she attack her body, but also she cleverly displaced her internal shame for yearning for her father's love onto her obesity. Her shame could now be something that was easily seen and felt and repaired quickly, once it took care of extinguishing her sexual feelings. She was now safe from her father, but not from her hidden and exciting shame. Since then she has thwarted any attempts to love a man but can allow sexual thoughts of fantasy men and their body parts. She can fill the room with her adolescent squeals of excitement at seeing an actor's rear end and how it turns her on. She remained a virgin until age 42, with her passionate exciting feelings attached to the Omnipotent Child that she will never give to a man or to her lust. Shame will conquer her and all the men. I was the recipient of her exciting feelings of disgust and denigration of my talents. I was the jackass. There was always something exciting when she went after me, and we would try to talk about that, with little result. Her complaints felt like foreplay between us.

To deal with the increasing relationship with me and the group, she took to an older man in her firm and developed a titillating asexual relationship with him. He was her boss. She would act like the little girl, and he would read her night-time stories. They would travel on trips together but play again like adolescents, with some exciting touching but clear boundaries. Her shame was that he was married, but she would never break up his family. This was a very meaningful relationship for her, which I didn't interfere with. She needed to let herself love a father who felt safe but had some early excitement in the relationship. She was now more ready for a healthier relationship.

Over time in the group, she had let herself get into a real relationship that unfortunately didn't go well, and now she is back trying to see if she will try again. She had sex, and was turned on by his rear end, but didn't feel the joy that she thought she should feel. These involvements were supported by the group, and the women made many efforts to be encouraging, like her mother wasn't.

Her shame is lessened, and she has begun to appreciate the excitement in disarming the men, in being indifferent to me, and the loneliness that exists in her, as she has begun to identify with George in the group. She is finally appreciating the excitement in being her father, by coming in late and really not caring about her effect on the other group members. She then talked about the new house she bought, and how empty it is, and how big it is, and how she doesn't know what to fill it with, or whether she can fill it. The shame is being replaced with her profound sense of loneliness and her desire to be with someone as she is getting older. She is now for the first time beginning to appreciate how she has not worked as hard as she could have in the group, how she has treated the group the way her father treated everyone in the family, how she has kept herself lonely and isolated and angry at me and/or the group for pushing her to be more connected. As she has let herself become more connected to the group, I notice a major change in her affect with us—she is more relaxed, and she smiles a great deal. She connects, as if the healthy, positive affects were tied up in the excitement of the shameful angry father identification. She could never find a man as long she was the father. She talked, sadly and movingly, as she recalled how excited and pleased she was at rejecting all the men. She asked the group to forgive her and apologized to the group for coming so late and, more importantly, for enjoying it. She has grudgingly begun to accept the fact that her putting on weight in adolescence was a way to control her shameful desires to be closer, and to feel sexual and adored by her very charismatic, narcissistic, seductive father. She is now for the first time allowing herself to have a desire for real people. The only person she was ever able to have lust for was and is still a movie actor, but that was only a part-object—his ass. She has noticed a renewed respect for my talents, and how she was struck that she liked me and would want to work with me individually when she leaves the group.

As the passion of the shame recedes and comes to light and is experienced in the group, healthy desire begins to come forward, which leads in some cases to further regression to the older passionate shame, and in others to a powerful but scary step forward to embrace the desire. Here the leader has a lot to do with what happens next.

Harry

Harry is a man who has been suffused since early childhood with shameful and exciting sexual fantasies that at times controlled his life and made him feel less than a man. They have made him feel too small, too needy, and too anxious. These feelings have been his Omnipotent Child organizers for most of his adult life, married life, and professional life as well. His marriage was almost asexual for the first 15 years, before he started treatment. I also saw his wife first and she and I recommended that he come into one of my groups. His shame was connected to being aroused and was influenced by his being at home with his very attractive mother and her very sexual sisters. The sexual fantasies had to be out of the house and out of the family, into the unknown woman. Sex with his wife was too close to the sisters and the mother. This then spread to any form of excitement and the shame of being a successful man. His shame was also fostered by his internal perception of failure to interest his father and get him more active in his life. He has been able to do that with me through his weekly dreams, to which we both look forward. He was encouraged to express his desires to the women in the group, and did so reluctantly, but with less shame over time. He was plagued by bouts of anxiety he didn't understand. In the group, he became fascinated by the shoes of a very seductive group member, Myrna.

The task was to help him begin to appreciate his excitement in the shame of desiring his mother and her sisters, in the face of a very passive and uninspiring father, and how that became an organizing Passionate Bad Fit for him all his life. I would try to get him to look at the desires for women in the group, but he was rather adamant about defending against that excitement in the family. Then there was Myrna, who openly fought me and tried to get me to be vulnerable and acknowledge mistakes I made with her, which she was quite good at. In the face of my vulnerability toward Myrna, Harry was able to begin to experience sexual feelings toward her and deal with the anxiety and the excitement. He felt less shame about it and was able now to talk of a more healthy sexual relationship with his wife. He would bring in dreams of sexual encounters with other unknown women and also with Myrna. He became a more sexual member in the group and he was pleased, even though, as was pointed out to him recently, he missed Myrna opening and closing her legs in front of him. I missed it also. At the same time, he is acknowledging his shame for his father's lack of excitement and his passivity. This has been channeled through his anger and contempt for George and the way he does business. His oedipal shame is being resolved, and the new shameless desires are being explored in the group and being corrected internally and with the group as a whole.

He has started his own business and survived the adoption of a child with some handicaps. He was able to talk about his sexual desires for both his children and the shame connected with it and was able to understand that the shame was his reaction to his early dependent longings for both his mother and his father, neither of which was satisfied.

August and Lenore

August and Lenore are trying to move to a more romantic, safe, and exciting relationship with each other, as they have to rid themselves of the bad mother in their lives. They do this through their dreams of his rescuing her and at the same time finding her very exciting and sexy.

She prefers to remain in the prison of childhood, where her mother can kill her if she ever expresses a need or wish or romantic feeling toward her father or anyone in the family. Lenore tended to punish the men in her life when they rejected her or stopped loving her unconditionally. She would ensure the man's need for her through sex, which still left her at the mercy of abandonment and terror. The group helped her to try to escape the prison. We put Mother in the "fireplace." August stayed steady and decided not to leave as he had thought earlier. She is still terrified of her needs and ashamed of them. He is now dealing with his shame of needing his wife and Lenore in a romantic, caring, holding way. His mother was seductive at times, especially through their mutual passion for painting, which he still enjoys fleetingly. He married a woman who expressed his terror and shame of being left and not being the most important one. When he was 16, his mother abandoned the family and left a note that put the blame on him. His wife was in one of my groups for about three years prior to my seeing August.

Lenore and August sit next to each other in the group and clearly define themselves as a couple. Lenore and Meg make peace and begin to withdraw from their threatening and deadly rivalry, as Meg tries to have a baby on her own. Both Meg and Lenore begin to notice how excited they were and how the group was excited by their continual confrontations with each other. We couldn't wait for the two to go at each other. They did that with meanness, injury, contempt, and shame-inducing comments. It wasn't until they could appreciate that their backgrounds were quite similar. Both suffered at the hands of narcissistic mothers, one more subtle, the other more overt. They both couldn't sustain relationships and blamed themselves and their partners. Both were ashamed of their deep yearnings for a good mother. Both had trouble with being admired by me or letting themselves love me. Both acted as if I loved the other more than I loved them. Reluctantly, they admitted to the excitement they felt about their fights and how passionate their rivalry was, more so than being loved by me or the group or a good mother. The field is clear for all three of them and the triangular dilemma is in the process of being solved for the group, as well as for them. Their coupling, which was encouraged by me and the group, highlighted the above positions and helped to clarify their rivalry and the resolution of that experience. Meg was able to find Bill in the group, an older man who really liked her and found her sexy and exciting. They both could have men in the group.

In a dream, Lenore lets August hold her hand as she leaves the prison, and in another dream she is in a hospital and notices the hospital gown is open, and she exposes her genitals without shame or distress. August smiles at this remarkable exposure. In turn, he exposes his fears as a child, and how he triumphed over his fears by crawling through pipes, hiding in trees, and so on. He worked through his shame around his terrible alcoholic father by revealing his deep wishes to be held by the older man (Bill) in the group. He and Lenore are enjoying the new-found excitement without shame and guilt, and she has been able to let him go, to terminate from the group.

Beth

Beth and I have worked together for many years, in individual therapy and in two different groups, each reflecting crises in her life of impulsive decisions, infantile acting-out, and a strong willfulness about getting a job or changing her relationships. They have all led to difficult, painful, and stressful times in her life, moving into precarious financial and/or relationship vulnerability. Her hallmark was her pleasantness, her likeability, and her willfulness, and not heeding any advice or suggestions to change the outcome of her life choices. Her last experience was with her newest beau, an Iranian, who was an alcoholic handyman and someone she needed to bail out. She was in love and he gave her the attention she longed for, the closeness, and the need to feel desired and important. However, as the relationship continued, she became shamefully more aware of how he kept draining her resources, and she felt like a battered woman who kept going back for more loving and eventual impoverishment. Her family grew up in collective shame about their poverty. I would see her periodically as she worked her way through this new relationship, and eventually made disastrous financial decisions that took her close to the shameful poverty of her childhood.

She steadfastly refused to heed my warnings, advice, and caring about her decisions with this man. I asked her to rejoin my once-weekly group to see if we could avoid disaster.

In the group, she organized around periods of silence and then periods of stories of her attachment to this man. I was struck by how charged the atmosphere was around her stories, and how excited and aroused the group became, either in getting angry at her or in passionately trying to protect her. Meanwhile, her money has run out and she has to leave the group. It became real, for the first time, how she didn't listen to the advice, even though she felt close and trusting of me over time, because she needed to keep being in the shameful position and in attachment to the power of the excitement of the shame. She could finally understand her confusion about why she couldn't stop her behavior, but it was too little, too late.

Jerry

Jerry is an example of unintegrated, archaic self-ego, where he announces without shame how he comes late because he never got an alarm clock. He can yell at me all he wants because that is how he feels, right or wrong, but, since it is contained in the group, he continually thrives in his family and at his job. He slowly becomes aware of his need to be more mature. I have worked with Jerry for over thirty years, which can be described as the most exciting, crazy-making, roller-coaster ride that I have ever been on. Diagnostically he is seen as both borderline and bipolar, with significant needs to act out. He first came to treatment because he was fired from a teaching job due to alcoholism and disrespect of authorities. He left treatment many times. He was in analysis and eventually three different groups over this time. With each treatment module, he got better, more mature, and was able to stop drinking. He settled down with a good spouse, had a son whom he loves, and has had stable job security for many years. He returned this last time because of forced retirement. He was scared and didn't want to mess up his life.

Jerry lived in shame—his mother got rid of him and sent him to his grandmother, who sent him back at age 8 to his mother. His mother was overtly seductive, and he was both terrified and excited that they would have intercourse. Later, he did sleep with his father's second wife. His first marriage was a sham, but his second and present marriage has been quite good, except for a lack of sexual desire on his part. He hated his mother and never resolved his hate for her. His intense reactions to me and the group were always a byproduct of his earliest infantile injuries at the hands of his mother. He loved and hated me. He denounced me. He left me as he was left. He couldn't stand it, yet admired and craved it, being my longest patient, and when I added another long-time patient he again left quickly. Old injuries don't die easily, but we learned a lot about his denial of his sadness from his acting out and his hypomanic quips and broadsides at me and the group. We did get back to that sad little boy. He hated me for making him give up the excitement of his shame and face the sadness and regrets of his life. Jerry left his mark on the group and is still talked about often. He left the group feeling his pain of being abandoned, but he also left them with a powerful set of images of the excitement in the shame of their lives.

He told a story of rats invading his house. He was aware of the excitement in finding them, trying to kill them, and calling the exterminator, but after a while it became more burdensome to him and he had to actually kill one, which he described with great enthusiasm and in great, vivid detail. The group was asked to struggle with the rat inside of them. That led Andrew, a rather quiet new member, to talk about his imaginary pal, a bumblebee that would let him do whatever he wanted to do and stop all interferences from anyone who intruded. The group talked about the murderous impulses that lurked inside, demons that they lived with, and issues that shamefully they felt they had to live with. Jerry then gave a full disclosure about the rats and how clever they were, and how they prefer to trick you and hide from you, and also how they are like us in that they have paws that feel human. The group is still struggling with the hidden rats. The group still misses him, as I do as well.

This case throws much light on the realm of masochistic delight, as well as the repeated need to be victimized, and how living in shame can be one of the most powerful organizers in some people, how some people need to repeat and repeat their shameful experiences to stabilize their flawed identity and template of intimacies of childhood. Rather than trying to eliminate shame, we need to appreciate the need to keep repeating it as a source of stability, no matter how horrendous their experiences are.

We can recognize the reluctance of therapists to go after shame and its hidden excitement, rather than being in awe of its power and authority. We have to learn not to be so intimidated or shamed by their shame, as if it was a failure on our parts, and see that it is a source of great power in a powerful Passionate Bad Fit.

How does one show the archaic grandiose self and its transformation in the group? This leads to my concept of *bigness* and letting oneself be big.

1 Having big fantasies of each other in the group, like sexual and aggressive and yearning fantasies. Letting Jason want to crawl into Diana's lap; letting Alex know how his sarcasm and contempt are worthy of special applause; letting Alice yell at the group for encouraging her to be sexual and all the problems that it creates.

2 Helping them live with the Passionate Good Fits and deal with the loneliness and regrets that follow, like Kris crying that it is too late to have a child and how she robbed herself of that pleasure.

3 The therapist acknowledges his moments of shame, and how he or she manages to regulate and integrate them, like the therapist forgetting details of a patient's life, regretting how he couldn't stop a patient from marrying a borderline spouse, how ashamed and sad he was, how he thoroughly enjoyed Lacey announcing with bravado how she loves me. How uncomfortable Myrna made me feel

when she pointed out my transference responses. How I will admit to patients that I am arrogant and wonder why they can't take some of that for themselves, since that is why some of them decided to work with me, to see how comfortable I am with my own integrated narcissism. My shame via Myrna, and how long I kept her in the group, when I should have terminated the work.

Chapter 6

Shame and Narcissism

The true aims of narcissism are to find and reunite with an idealized object or ego ideal and also to experience autonomy, separation, identity uniqueness, grandiosity, perfection, and competence. Narcissism is in a bind. You cannot have both at once. The wish for merger can lead to shame, since you cannot do it alone. Shame seems to be embedded in all aspects of narcissism. Shame can also be defensive, to protect you from your own grandiosity and omnipotence. Shame is the irritant that leads to the disruption of the merged grandiosity of the mother–infant dyad. This rupture or misstatement leads to the formation, through the body, of a neuronal channel that gets lodged in the right cerebral hemisphere. This neuronal channel I have labeled the Passionate Bad Fit or the Omnipotent Child channel.

Origins of narcissism:

1 From where does the energy come to fuel the earliest aspects of grandiosity, or is it assumed to be part of the infantile toolbox? Kohut (1978, 1984) believes that the infant's loss and trauma lead to the fantasized archaic grandiosity and bliss. When that part of the archaic ego is ruptured, shame floods the system.
2 The grandiosity of the infant must be mirrored by the mothering figure, and they have to deal with their mutual excitement and perfection at that moment. Then life goes on. Injury happens. Ruptures occur. The perfection is damaged in both parties.
3 The energy comes from the mutual grandiosity and excitement located in that mix. Therefore, the soma must be involved as the source of that special energy supply. I assume that the body ego, the ego ideal, and the Omnipotent Child all reside in the tissues of the soma. The body, when excited, lays down neuronal channels that can supply the required energy. That allows the unhealthy narcissism, which is filled with shame as the irritant, to get embedded in the right cerebral hemisphere.
4 Do the new neuronal channels carry the shame that led to the ruptures, like the Omnipotent Child? Yes, since the shame starts the whole process going by causing the rupture that keeps the grandiosity in check but also adds another dimension—the Omnipotent Child.

DOI: 10.4324/9781032705835-8

5 How does an oyster make a pearl? It needs an irritant to do it, to create the compound that coats the oyster and shell that allows the pearl to form. Not all oysters make pearls; not all children become narcissistic personalities. The irritant, I propose, is shame, which causes the start of the formation of the pearl, i.e., the formation of the Omnipotent Child. The pearl is the unique grandiosity of the infant.

6 As a result, shame carries not only the energy and the process of the irritant that leads to ruptures but also must then have its own need for excitement and durability to be so important a process in the development of the human condition.

7 Shame becomes a stabilizer of the Passionate Bad Fit identity. Shame then becomes a comfort, like a lap to many patients, but also costs an exorbitant price to stay stabilized. Therefore, many seek out the experience of shame as a stabilizer of an early somatically bound identity.

How and where does narcissism start? First is the baby–mother dyad, all enveloped within their shared, merged grandiosity. The grandiosity is in the infant's toolkit and is present at birth. Then there is a rupture in that merger, and shame enters the picture. This rupture then sends the infant on the road to recover his omnipotence. The archaic grandiosity (Kohut, 1978, 1984) takes over and the merger is temporarily stabilized. This gets repeated often throughout the first year. There is rupture, then merger, in the first year of life, as the dyad seeks common ground and less ability to hurt each other's grandiosity. At this point, my theory of the Omnipotent Child and the Passionate Bad Fit takes over the discourse and becomes the substance of both my technique and theory of my group therapy experiences.

Chapter 7

Healthy Desire and Aliveness

The Group's Power to Work through the Passion in Shame

What is the Omnipotent Child? It is that part of the body ego that holds the residuals of all the earlier misattunements in the pre-verbal state of being. It is fueled by the somatic arousals that accompany these early misattunements, which help lay down neuronal tracks that contain the Passionate Bad Fit, and tend to stabilize identity and templates of intimacy for the newborn. There is the potential at each succeeding phase of development for the Omnipotent Child to be reinvigorated, and the neuronal tracks to be more stabilized. The need to repeat is not just to master the injury, but as Kernberg (2001), Cohen, 2000, and others suggest, it is a way to stabilize the earliest identity and templates of intimacy. This also includes the need to live in shame or be miserable with shame.

So many patients enter treatment because their excitement and passion has led them to wrong places, wrong decisions, and bad relationships. Some enter because they can't have desire or passion. I call these relationships *Passionate Bad Fits*. The passion they are feeling is the wrenching agony and misery of their lives and, in particular, the trapped, victimized feelings. Desireless people live in the agony of missed opportunities, regret, and feelings of failure over a lifetime. What brings them into treatment? They can't deal with it anymore; relationships have broken, jobs have been lost, their children have acted out, and are in trouble. They have tried different treatments and have noticed that their great empty halls are still not filled. What kind of passion am I talking about? The passion is intertwined with somatic arousal and shame. The passion in the hidden excitement of surviving in the original basic somatic identity, no matter the cost to themselves or others. This is where Morrison (1989) talks about the intertwining of narcissism and shame. Inherent in the Passionate Bad Fit is shame. How did it get there? Alonso and Rutan (1993) describe how shame arises from the earliest autistic or pre-oedipal stage, thus making it one of our primal affects.

Shame occurs when the infant's body is not properly soothed and maintained by the mothering figure. The infant's body experiences a failure, and the early origins of failure form the nuclei of shame in the body ego. Klein (1946) tried to talk about these early, pre-verbal but not neurologically dead moments. The wiring is already in motion to develop the proper channels of safety and pleasure. The infant's earliest pre-verbal somatic desires have a powerful effect on the laying

DOI: 10.4324/9781032705835-9

down of neuronal channels in the right brain and impact on the development of the neuro-endocrine systems. The early power of these desires and the potential for failure are the origins of the Omnipotent Child in the body ego, the first and last ego we live in.

How do we take these concepts and translate them into effective group therapy? I have set up a construct of the Omnipotent Child in the group, with the therapist acting as the mother of symbiosis (Mahler, 1968). I have constructed a developmental model that the group seemed to go through in many iterations.

1 The fit, the lap, and the symbiotic mother.
2 The body and separation–individuation—hatching.
3 Sexuality, ambiguity, and safe harbors.
4 The working-through phase.

As a therapist, my basic belief is that all the members are babies, and I am the most important member in the group. I then act accordingly and interfere when group members try to talk to each other. I bring them back to me and deal with all the reactions attendant to that approach. I work with each to help them tell the stories of the preverbal times in their life. The group complains about my position yet coalesces around the storytelling of the most difficult period in their lives. No one has wanted to hear their stories, even though they repeat them incessantly. People tell their stories in all kinds of ways—some through music, paintings they love, or body movements like the rooster and the guy who called to complain the fee was too high, to tell me how colicky he was as an infant.

Through this model, the earliest moments of shame and failure take over the group dynamic. The therapist's lap is introduced to the group, received with great derision and mocking. Then they realize that they never had a safe, loving, nurturing lap in their life and how their own lap is not nurturing either, and they see how they relate to others as either the ultimate rescuer or the indifferent, self-involved, and conflict-avoidant lap in the room. How they relate to the offer of the lap tells a great deal about the corruption in their normal, healthy desires, and henceforth shame has to be hidden in those desires.

To be discussed later is how the shame gets there. Using the model of projective identification, the mothering or fathering figure projects his or her failure into the most vulnerable object, the baby, then the child, and then the adult. When we see our patients, they have mostly been invaded by the shame of the parents and they carry it with great distinction and heroism.

Kohut (1978, 1984) believed that the infant deals with present and eventual losses and trauma through fantasies of archaic grandiosity and bliss. When there is corruption in this magnificent state of being, shame floods the system. Since these disruptions are centered in somatically aroused Passionate Bad Fits, the shame is somatically aroused and takes on a pattern of excitement and heroism fueled by the archaic grandiosity. When I point out that heroism is the problem, the group usually colludes against my lack of empathy for their heroism. How could I be so disdain-ful of this? I let them know how powerful it must feel to be that special child who could hold on to their shame with such magnificence. The heroic position of the shame carrier is their Omnipotent Child or Passionate Bad Fit.

They will also arrange events that keep the shame alive, one way or another. There are people who live in shame, and there are groups who live in shame, as well as leaders who also live in shame.

After working that through, we are left with the ultimate dilemma. How do you put the shame that you have carried back into the people who put it in you? Is it necessary to do anything with the acknowledged shame that you carry? Should you just put it down and move on with your life? Should you forgive and be willing to carry the sadness rather than the shame? Is acknowledging the shame enough for the desired character change and thus major changes in the patient's life? Will dealing with shame lead to major changes and risks that the group and the patients signal as a move toward the Passionate Good Fit? Can the group and the patients tolerate the existential angst of periods of a lost identity? Can they uncover the hid-den excitement in prolonging shame?

How do we recognize the impact shame has had on a patient's and group's re-lationships, desires, and internal sense of self and identity and the templates of intimacy? How do we know that shame is operating in the group, in the patient, and in the therapist? The first thing to notice is how the group deals with desires. When shame is early in one's life, desire and passion become embedded in the Passion-ate Bad Fit. As a result, there is a profound early corruption of the neurobiologi-cal substrate of desire. It is filled with too much aggression, failure, neediness, or sexuality to be able to be regulated in a healthy way. That becomes the major work of the group.

The second thing to notice is how they respond to the offer of the therapist's lap. This tells a great deal about the depth of the injuries in childhood and how the no-tion of a safe and secure lap is so foreign to them and terrifying of the thought of a good fit, since that would be a betrayal of the Omnipotent Child. One can sense when the group is putting their shame into the therapist. They do this by coming late, acting out, becoming stubborn, or living in self-righteous indignation. The therapist, at this point, must pay special attention to her own acting out the shame that is put into her by the group.

Buddy is an example of how and what to do with the knowledge that you have been carrying your parents' shame and humiliation as parents and as people. It took Buddy about two years of work in the group to even notice that his depression, lack of desire, low motivation for fun, low self-esteem, and strong feelings that no woman would find him exciting were symptoms of shame. The relief and indignity of naming his symptoms as shame got him to start questioning his early life. He struggled with this, with the group's help in identifying their own shame and how ubiquitous it appears.

Buddy then had to deal with how to get rid of it. I took the position that you need to try to put it back into the parents and/or see where it is in the group. "Who is putting shame into you here now?" This was incredible to him and the group. He found Holly, who had clearly let the group know that she thought quite poorly of men and that she was the best man in the group. Since Buddy was a bit more freed up about his shame, he was able to notice how attractive Holly was. He talked openly about this, and Holly talked about how attractive he was and how it might be nice if they were together. She shared a dream where she was seducing him by moving closer to him, and he didn't respond to that dream in the group immediately. She shortly thereafter asked the group's permission to go to a training group run by a therapist who she thought was gorgeous and still continue in the group. The group was excited for her except for Buddy, who at that point could not put his feelings into words.

Buddy felt himself withdrawing and feeling alone and isolated, like he used to feel before joining the group. He was able to see, with the group's help, how Holly had shamed him and how he quickly accepted the shame, but now wanted to give it back to her. He got angry directly with her about her other snipes at his maleness and how she dumped him for this other leader. I pointed out that the injury is quite powerful, since his father also dumped him for another man. Holly then had to struggle with how she shames men as a way to not notice how ashamed she felt as a little girl, surrounded by brothers and feeling unloved and unlovable. There was no place for her in the family. "I was an ugly child with unmanageable hair, and I wasn't nice to people." She had made great strides in these feelings through her 4-year-old daughter, who she was raising herself, and her feeling that she could take shots at me about my decisions and how we could deal with each other about that. Instead of anger and hurt, she was feeling long-overdue sadness for the little girl inside of herself and was trying to let her out in the group. She had let herself be more vulnerable to Buddy and to her own sadness and shame that she desired so much more from her father and continually failed herself.

Buddy went to visit his father at the father's request, and nothing happened that he wished would happen. He complained about how the trip cost him a fortune with no gains. Father still would not talk about how he shut him out of his life. The next week he went again looking to keep alive the Omnipotent Child, so he won't get on with his life without shame as the organizer, worrying and stewing over his father's intransigence. He also called his 74-year-old mother and said no to her request that he join her at the beach before he went away. He was learning to say no and to say yes. He was beginning to enjoy life and the window of desire was opening for him.

Part 3

Anger and Aggression

In this section, the group's plunge into anger and rage is explored, and attempts at solutions and understanding and the role of the therapist are discussed. Ways to understand the powerful affects in the context of the group's Passionate Bad Fit and, at the same time, to locate the group's shame are addressed. The future of the group is on the line. The actions and behaviors of the therapist are seen through the lens of his own shame.

DOI: 10.4324/9781032705835-10

Chapter 8

Anger in Groups

The literature on anger in groups is sparse. Its role in either fermenting growth or regression is still an issue among group therapists. Does the power and expression of anger and the underside of disappointments in not being able to reunite with earlier imagined and somatically felt oneness and therefore grandiosity reflect the health in groups? Nitsun (1996) specifically focuses on the group's anger at the therapist and the work that is needed to get done. Their wish to destroy the therapist and the anti-group process is slow to build up but once it becomes conscious and in the group it can be very destructive. In one of my examples, I describe a group that nearly unraveled when intense near psychotic rivalry and envy took over. Nitsun (1996) describes some destructive forces that tend to make it possible for the anti-group process to develop. There is fear of exposure, distrust of the group, a frustration of narcissistic needs, and the resultant feelings of shame and anger that they have not been seen and nourished by the group as mother. There is also genuine rivalry and envy and competition that mostly leads to shame and humiliation or grandiosity that can be fed by the concomitant shame.

I encourage anger in the group when I repeatedly announce at the beginning of our work together that I am the most important person in the room. Their narcissism is right in the room embedded in the therapist. They do not like it but admit that they have already endowed me with magical powers and narcissistic grandiosity. There is again relief that these feelings can be talked about without shame and fear. When they see me own my narcissism without shame, anxiety, or fear, they begin to feel that maybe they can own their own narcissism through the work in the group. They, for the most part, have rarely had the experience of healthy narcissism in them and in their families. It is through the therapist's healthy narcissism that one can look at the shame that intensifies and organizes the unhealthy narcissism. Therapists must come clean and divulge to the group when they feel shame or act in a shameful manner. Rarely do therapists discuss, much less announce their importance in the group. Therapists then put themselves at a disadvantage when they are surprised that the group wants to overthrow them, or demands that they be the objects of desire or scapegoating, and, most importantly, can take what the group can dish out, via their anger, sadness, silence, or negativity. Therapists must

DOI: 10.4324/9781032705835-11

let themselves be big and hold what is in the group, including the shame and grandiosity. Groups form to work with you, the specific therapist. The therapist must have an ability to be "therapeutically aggressive." It is not easy to train therapists to allow themselves, in the context of the transference, to be the bad mother or father and not overcome their therapeutic skill through empathy. They sometimes use empathy as a way to avoid the bruising battles that are inside most of our patients, and ourselves. As a result, the work suffers and the potential for healthy narcissism to be explored gets lost. For the therapist, healthy narcissism allows availability of the approximate degree of empathy that he feels the patients need. Most therapists do not assume that it is the willingness to do battle and confront in a "therapeutic aggressive manner" (Stillerman, 2023, private conversation) the hidden issues that keep the conflicts front and center in their lives, which allows them to become more conscious and more available to the patient and the group.

The anger gives us a chance to get early information on the misattunements in the early nonverbal time in the patient's life. When the anger is encouraged as a tool by the therapist and group members for further development of their story that must be told, there is a marked relief to know that this anger has been inside of them for as long as they can remember and belongs to that preverbal period of life. That will take time to consider, but it quiets them down, they say, and makes them feel safer. The anger then is quite progressive and important in their own future development and in understanding their powerful silence and how much harm it has done to them. A patient, after many years of treatment, finds it almost unbearable to speak the unspoken and still suffers from a lack of desire for a healthy romantic attachment.

The anger in patients can be detected by their uncommon silence, agitation, or erratic behavior, and in their coming and going in the group. I use anger in the group as a hallmark for where the group is developmentally. If there is no aggression in the group for a period of time, the therapist has to begin to wonder whether the aggression is covered with shame, profound disappointment, and sadness and therefore has to remain hidden. The therapist must also consider his own anger at the group or at particular members of the group. He may be joining the group in choosing shame and silence, rather than speaking the unspeakable. The therapist may be as uncomfortable with his aggression and his fear that he or she will lose the ability to empathize and be the parent they did not have. Therapists are not being taught how to be therapeutically aggressive and still have empathy for the patients. They certainly need to be.

The aggression in the opening phases of the group has to do with my encouraging them to see me as the mother of symbiosis. The earliest misattunements come flooding out and the anger and shame and loss are co-mingled with mixed emotions of trying to attach to me as the mother, and at the same time flee from her. They cannot trust me, nor should I trust them. Therapists have rarely talked about how the group at the beginning should and will not trust each other until you discuss the basic distrust that unites the group. Basic trust hopefully comes later in the work.

It is highly unusual today for therapists to talk openly about how they do not trust the group. If only the infant could say to the mothering figure,

> I sadly do not trust that you will really pay enough attention to me, feed me when I need to be fed, hold me as needed, and still make me feel that I am the most magnificent child you ever had and you are the most magnificent mother that I ever had.

A very wonderful and admired senior therapist and I have a battle about how much trust you should have in the group doing its work. He thinks that, in time, the group will do the work, and he is more passive and curious about how the group functions. Needless to say, I am on the other side. I really do not trust the group at the beginning and do not expect them to do the work on their own without acting out to tell their story. They all need to tell their story in their own way. Therefore, I am much more active and powerful and put myself in the center of the group by announcing that I am the most important person in the group at that moment. Scapegoating is common in the early stages of the group, as it is in the later stages of triangles. There is always a loser in a triangle. The therapist has to make sure that patients do not become the object of either hatred or longed-for desire and shame, and the leader must assume that responsibility. The anger also marks where the hidden sadness lies and who carries it for the group. Inevitably, a patient will rise to the occasion and play out being the receptacle for the aggression, sadness, and shame for the group. They must be protected by the therapist. I will now proceed to give an example of aggression in the group and how we deal with it.

> In an ongoing weekly group, there were two woman who were trying to kill (or be killed by) each other. I had seen Robin in the past and she was married to a man who, in disassociate states, clearly wanted to kill her. She sensed that, but really couldn't allow the implications. She returned to this group, wanting to divorce her husband. She had powerful feelings of injustice around her bi-racial adopted kids. She always sought empathy in the group, but tended to decline it when she got it. She had been very connected to me throughout, and I to her. I really felt her injured life, from her childhood on, and found her to be a highly valuable member of the group. She spoke the truth, was unafraid to mix it up, and could be loving, caring, and provocative at various times in the group.
>
> Rhonda was the other combatant in this mix. She was a very well-put-together, attractive woman, who was also in the field, and who came to the group to work on becoming more comfortable with anger in herself and in her patients. She got much more than she bargained for. Her entry was marked by jealous and envious reactions from Robin and others, because she wasn't in an acute state of distress and looked too pretty to be part of the group. I didn't know whether she could tolerate the group's barrage, and I had to do intense work to point out their envy.

I also made clear that Robin's anger toward Haren was actually for me. *Why would I bring Rhonda into the group? Why aren't we enough for you? How dare there be another baby, much less an adorable one who will sweep me off my feet, something that these women didn't feel from either of their parents.* I wanted the men in the group to do more work to help me keep her in the group. They did reluctantly, as they enjoyed the constant struggle between the women as a defense against exposing their sexual feelings toward her and their competitive feelings as well. The men tried to stay asexual for long stretches of this group. Their competition with me felt too difficult to tackle, even when talked about.

All of us, the men, the women, and me, all added to the outbursts between Robin and Rhonda in the following months of the group. We all allowed and encouraged them to relive the earliest painful and shameful attachments in their lives. As I have noted before, patients need to feel healthier, and have more good, caring objects inside of them to be able to allow themselves to regress to the most shameful moments in their lives. Robin insisted that she could not work with Rhonda because she was hurtful and aggressive, and had fooled everyone. "She is like my mother," Rhonda would always say. "Yes, I can be manipulative and angry, like in that fight with my husband." But Robin was not seduced by that. At one point, Robin spoke, angrily and sadly, of how in the group she felt psychotic at times, as if there were an evil presence in her that was tormenting her and not letting her be civil to anyone. I was quite concerned that this psychotic core had been there all the time, and we hadn't been able to expose and understand it. This information came out after she divorced her (at times) psychotic husband, who felt that he needed to plunge a knife into her to love her better. She used to work for a company that found and exploded war bombs in the Balkans. Rhonda was terrified of having temper tantrums in adult life, as she did as a kid and was sent to her room for punishment. Rhonda wanted to scream at Robin, but felt too restrained, but as she sat and listened to Robin's rants against her, Robin became Rhonda's highly critical father, and her fury at me for not protecting her from Robin got verbalized—a Hobson's choice for me and the group. I waited and hoped that someone from the group would rise to the occasion and try to make peace, but it didn't happen. We obviously needed more fireworks before we could start the empathetic resolution of the co-created regressive attachments and Passionate Bad Fit disorders in their lives in the past and present in the room.

The tension waxed and waned for the next couple of weeks, and I saw each one separately in individual consultations that they both asked for. I tried to convince each of them to stay and work it out. They were dubious, but I wasn't. I had been through this before in another group, and I knew that both parties felt strong attachments to me, which would carry us through to the resolution.

In the last session the rage and hurt and fear erupted. Robin was uneasy, and I could see her fidgeting, and I felt that her rage and need to leave the group were strong. A group member asked her what was wrong. She started screaming that Rhonda's presence in the room was wrong, that she could not live here with her. She knew she wanted to kill her, and she couldn't talk about anything else in her life, because she was terrified of Rhonda. Rhonda sat motionless and started to cry. I felt helpless and scared; I had a father who could rage as well. Robin then said that she was so sad for me, she loves me and she knew I had her best interests at heart, but I was stuck between them. She had to leave anyway, since I wouldn't kick her out—she knew I would never kick her out if the roles were reversed. No matter that Rhonda had shown more real anger in the group, had become more real and admitted that she could be seductive to avoid anger, like demanding that the group not let this fight just be between them. Rhonda yelled at the group that she needed them to own what is the group's. Robin was unmoved and still convinced that Rhonda wanted to kill her. A group member said that she didn't believe that Rhonda wanted to kill her. Robin calmed down briefly, since she truly respected that member. I turned to Rhonda and said, "I hope you can understand that I have to work with Robin right now, since I don't want her or you to leave this group and want both of you to stop living in the trauma, and begin to grieve it, and feel the abject loneliness and sorrow of childhood and of your adult life."

Someone suggested they needed more empathy for each other. I said they needed more empathy for themselves, not for each other. "Your empathy for your parents led both of you to hold on to the traumas that belonged to them." I said that they deserved our admiration and applause in exposing the rage, hurt, sadness, and pain that had lived in everyone in the group. I commented about how sad it was for Robin to feel that, not only did her mother not want her, but also wanted to kill her to avoid her total lack of maternal identification. The group had to begin to find enough empathy in themselves to quell the fury and fear of their traumas. "All of you in this group have had early traumas, and still are reluctant to name it and to empathize with your hurt, which you were not responsible for. Robin and Rhonda have shown the way to expose the traumas of early life, and the shame that you all carry for your parents to be the special loved ones. The traumas are in the group room now, and have to be addressed, so neither Robin nor Rhonda have to leave this group. The hidden trauma has to be exposed together, and be replaced by sorrow, sadness, more empathy for yourselves, and hopefully for others and a new lease on the way forward to Passionate Good Fits."

Chapter 9

Aggression

In my theory of the Passionate Bad Fit, and the Omnipotent Child, the therapist, at the beginning of the group, is the most important person in the room. He takes on the role of the symbiotic mother. The patients are all considered newborns. In this beginning phase, the therapist intervenes to understand some early symbolic meanings in their narrative. They therefore relate to the therapist as if they were in their original dyad. The therapist's symbolic lap is a constant presence throughout the group experience. The Passionate Bad Fit arises from the somatic sensory experiences of misattunements in the pre-verbal period of life. Those highly charged somatic experiences lay down neuronal pathways in the right brain. This Passionate Bad Fit or Omnipotent Child has enormous power over defining one's identity, the nature of attachments, and object ties, as well as their relationship to inner conflicts. The Omnipotent Child is the container of all the early misattunements in the child's life. The work of group therapy is to be able to move from a Passionate Bad Fit to a Passionate Good Fit. To do that, emotional strength and maturity are built slowly. This leads to the group being able to ultimately betray their original attachments. Aggression is present from the onset, as the early longings for the good mother lead to hurt and loss.

Lenny and August's Struggle

Here is an example of a once-a-week group in its fourth year together, where I saw some of the patients in individual therapy as well.

August, a teacher, was healthy enough to finally get in touch with his rage at his abusive father. He wished he had never been born. August was an outstanding member of the group, who was respected and highly esteemed. When Lenny, an engineer, came into the group, August treated Lenny, with the help of some other members, with contempt. Lenny came to the group to deal with his difficulty in handling his anger. Lenny was an attractive man, who acted at first as if this was a group just for him. His narcissism showed early. Lenny was puzzled by August's attack on him, while August was in his glory cutting Lenny down to size. I said to the group, "August couldn't bear living in the Passionate Good

DOI: 10.4324/9781032705835-12

Fit with the group. There is another narrative in him that Lenny has stirred up. And at this time, he can't find the painful memories to put into words, but he will. It is so important that this battle can be engaged in the group." This battle of August bullying Lenny continued for many weeks and months. Insults were hurled at Lenny, and his pain showed. Lenny wanted the group to protect him from August. Lenny wanted out of the group. I suggested, "August has stirred up some very painful memories of how scared you were as a kid without your father's protection from your sadistic, sexually stimulating mother. Now we can help you put those fears in a different context."

Lenny saw the group as his impotent father who never protected him from mother. Attempts to calm them and to minimize the damage being done to both of them didn't work. From time to time, Lenny burst forth with abusive comments to August. August got furious at me and demanded that I make Lenny leave the group because he was too abusive. I said, "Lenny is not leaving, and neither are you. We are going to deal with both your rages, and figure this out in this group." The group was quiet, or commented that they hoped this fight would stop. "This battle has touched all of you. Many of you have described being abused and abusive." The group came to life and was able to identify with the combatants. I felt that both men still might leave the group and a part of me wished they would.

Lenny finally stopped bullying August and was able to express his needs to the group. He was so lonely, sad, and angry growing up, so unprotected and hated. These things have plagued Lenny his whole life. I felt the whole group was at risk and I reminded the group that the struggle between August and Lenny was in all of us. The fight between August and Lenny then shifted dramatically. Lenny, at an early age, was sexually abused by his sadistic mother. He continued this Passionate Bad Fit in his life and in the group with August. Intimacy for both of them meant abuse that was overwhelming and over-stimulating. I then said, "It's easier for both of you to live in your Passionate Bad Fits than to come into my lap. I want you both to try to imagine how you could be held in my lap as infants. My lap can handle your aggression as well as your loneliness and sadness. Please tell us when it gets too stimulating in here." August intends to enliven the "dead fucking group" to remind himself of his old identity of living with overstimulation.

August then was able to step back from his need to abuse Lenny, and began to sob and be enraged at the same time. He was furious at me for letting Lenny enter and remain in the group. He would scream and sob that he hated me for not wanting to hear about how crazy and ugly he could be. I acknowledged that I did have a hard time really hearing the depth of his despair as a little boy. I was torn between whom to protect, and to whom to listen. August screamed as he said, "You know I care about you. We've worked together for so long. I don't want to put you through this. I know how hard this is for you. But I have to leave the group. I can't stay in this group with him in it. It brings out the worst in me and I hate myself." "No," I responded, "you hate your sadistic father and hate when you become him and Lenny becomes little August, overwhelmed by you as your sadistic father. Now we know what your father was really like, and the horror you had to live with in that family." This also, unconsciously resonated with Lenny and his fear of his mother and his own fears as a kid.

I said, "It is okay that you scared us, since it may have been your only way to bring this narrative to the group." August calmed down after that. The group began to recall their own traumas that had not been exposed the way August's and Lenny's were. August still took shots at Lenny, but the steam had gone out of it, and he talked about his life outside of the group, which he hadn't done for a while. Lenny grew more comfortable with his own aggression and could deal with his sadness about his mother. They both tried to fantasize getting in my lap, being either rocked or lying on my chest and being held. They both wanted to know that they could leave the lap when they had enough. The group survived and so did I. I became much more aware of the traumas in my own life, and how I dealt with them through humor, sarcasm, and perpetual fights with my brother.

It is hard to give up the Passionate Bad Fit identity and be disloyal. The undoing is to merge again with the oppressor and give your shame to someone else in the group. Lenny did not accept it and they fought over it. Life is not as heroic in the Passionate Good Fit.

Chapter 10

Case Examples of Fighting in Groups

There has been very little written about specific examples of battles or fights between the therapist and the group members, or between group members. I would speculate that since the goal is to put thoughts and feelings into words, not action, fighting would be seen as a potential failure of the goal of prohibiting action. Fighting could also be seen by the therapist and the group community as a failure of leadership, or the uncovering of the shameful intensity of narcissism.

The advent of intersubjectivity, the notion that the therapist and the group collude to form the nucleus of some of the traumatic events in the members' and the group's life, makes acting out more reasonable as a therapeutic model. Therapists now feel more able to expose their own personal lives and to make themselves more real and empathetic. There is great danger in that. How much should the therapist engage in playing out the members' drama? How much should therapists expose their own history to assuage the members and give them the sense that someone understands and knows what they have been through? In many of these situations, therapists lose the ability to listen for the orchestral music, rather than the cymbal clash. They give up an important function by not choosing listening and holding over the dramatic moment of empathy and closeness.

There is no reason, therefore, that a therapist and group member should expose their frustrating anger toward each other. The therapist must own up to his role in enabling this situation to take place and to develop into and reach its emotional high. That could be represented through mutual melancholia, helplessness, hopelessness, rage, sexual desires, or shame, as well as rageful fantasies.

In my theory and technique, the therapist announces, at the beginning, that he is the most important person in the group and acts accordingly. This, in itself, can lead to any of the above feeling states, as well as a confluence of competition and envy and the need to dethrone the therapist. The therapist must be able to hold all these conflicted and high-intensity emotions in his body and mind to enable the members to tell the stories of their early wordless years.

With this background, it is not farfetched to imagine that, at the beginning, when there is "fight, flight, or freeze," there will be attention to the interactions between the therapist and the new member, so as to examine the early misattunements that the member is still carrying, usually in his or her body, with concurrent emotional states.

DOI: 10.4324/9781032705835-13

Each part of the developmental phases that the members and group go through will have moments of potential rage, aggression, and hostility toward the therapist toward other group members, and ultimately toward themselves. Fighting and mutual frustration can drag on through many different phases of development, or just be acute and highlight traumatic events or shameful moments in their lives.

The therapist may feel that his narcissistic grandiosity is being attacked, disrespected, or demeaned. The member may experience the therapist's narcissism as overbearing, shaming, or humiliating, and unable to be talked about rationally in the group. The therapist may feel that the member is trying to destroy the group, and therefore must be expelled. The therapist is highly susceptible to the stimulus of the member's history and its potential to elicit very painful and shaming moments in the therapist's life. The therapist can be overcome with desire and then allow shame to take over his rational thoughts. He may be subject to bouts of unhealthy narcissism driven by shame. When that occurs, this unhealthy narcissism is filled with excess aggression, revengeful fantasies, regressive toxic mergers, and the belief that he is licensed to put these feelings into action.

The fight that ensues allows both protagonists to recreate powerful moments in their lives, which were either played out or suppressed. The fight is an attempt on their parts to return to homeostasis and recover from their respective regressions into the Passionate Bad Fit. They both must acknowledge that and then they can begin to analyze the fight and speculate about how to proceed.

The Patient with the Hoodie

Gail (who I have described elsewhere in the book) and I struggled throughout her work, and she was one of the more difficult members to work with. She wore a hoodie to hide herself. Her shame was profound, and she held on to it tightly for dear life. It was her only attachment to her parents. She presented as if she had no desire for anything, any work or relationships (including her husband), except with her dog, who gave her unconditional love and loyalty with very few demands. She took this for granted and never fully appreciated his love for her.

Everything else was too hard for her. She refused to look for a job, even though she was very well trained for many positions. She relied on her husband, who was having trouble with his teaching career. She ultimately would acquiesce to his needs but did not treat him with the respect and dignity that he deserved. Her neediness spilled out all over the place, as well as her hidden shame, self-degradation, and failure. She believed that she was a failed child and adult with no escape. She was angry at the world most of the time. She was the one who did not get better in the group. "How magnificent this must be for you," I said,

> as you stake out the lonely, sad, hopeless, failed, Passionate Bad Fit identity. You came by it honestly, and I understand that. You tell your story well. But now we have to try to help you face up to the shame that drives the old identity. We have our work ahead of us, but I would not have taken you into this group if I thought you could not work with us.

Gail very quickly exposed her anger at a few members, at the same time frustrating the group's attempts to help her understand why she would not find a job. She complained of lack of money constantly and had to borrow from her mother to pay my bill.

Her entitlement really pissed me off. She reminded me of my older brother and his entitlement to treat people sadistically and still expect his ring to be kissed. She would openly reject any advice from the other members, especially me. She thought I should understand her plight, help her get a job, and leave her alone. "Do not investigate me," she would say. I would say, "There is a need for you to remain a hidden mystery. Who was a mystery to you growing up?" She at times would respond that her older sister was healthier and got the spotlight, while she felt like the adopted one and the forgotten one. I told her,

> It must be quite difficult to hold your own with all these women in the group. Your envy and shame at not being as good as them must be so hurtful to you. It seems your only defense against the inherent shame you carry for this failure is to act infantile and abusive and threatening, to conquer your internal shame.

After she told me to go to hell, the group tended to confirm what I had said but felt I was too harsh. I concurred and apologized to her and the group. She laughed as if she had "got" me. I would point out to her, when she would rebuff me and others in the group and rip into them (including me) for investigating her motives, that she certainly was not hidden any longer.

Gail began to join forces with some other angry women in the group, and there were times when I felt overwhelmed and needed supervision, since it felt like the group was out of control, particularly the women. I asked one woman to leave when she began exhibiting paranoid symptoms, which created quite a mess in the group. The men felt paralyzed and stunned by the aggression in the room.

I felt paralyzed, fearful, and inadequate to deal with her paranoia and the increasing rage in the group, where Gail was one of the leaders. I did manage to say to Gail, "I guess you've finally found a passionate job." My narcissism and investment in the health of this group was on the line. I was injured, bereft, lost, and filled with shame. I had to figure out how I was going to think about this rage, regression, and sadistic behavior toward the group members. This must have been the rageful shame that her stepfather put into Gail. The intensity threatened the very existence of the group and its safety and reliability. Some threatened to leave, Gail being one of them, and this threatened the ending of the group.

I usually could put these dramatic moments into the context of the group's reactions to my loss of power and taking on the shame of the hoodie. We were living in a collective sense of failure to protect and prevent the paranoid thoughts projected on one of the members, Robin. I cared a great deal about Robin and so did the group. She was riding high, had found a man she loved, but had to undo the recent successes of living in the Passionate Good Fit. This new healthy identity was fragile and could easily be undone. She needed to gather her courage and strength and deal with the disloyalty of trying to leave the toxic merger with her borderline and fragile mother. The undoing was organized around her envy, rage, and anxiety about not being my favorite woman in the group. She focused all her anxieties and intense feelings on a new, attractive, female member who had entered the group. These intense feelings led her to re-merge with her borderline mother as a way not to leave her and not to feel disloyal.

We all suffered greatly from these unconscious actions and feelings. They were beyond interpretation; Sue held fast to her fragile wish for me to get rid of this member. "She doesn't belong here. She's too healthy for this group. You only want her to be here so you can have sexual fantasies about her." The group then took sides, with the men trying to understand the women's envy and rivalry. It was like nothing they had experienced before. They said it was too open: "We try to keep it in the ballgame." I countered, "We are as open now as you are tackling on the field or beating out a competitor in the office." This was an eye-opener for the men.

The women all joined the new member, Rhonda, and showed their new-found aggression to others: to some of the men, but especially to me. One man, quivering, told Gail that she played with her pencil in such a way that he was terrified that she was going to come over and stab him. Gail, for the first time, was confronted with her naked aggression as he took the pencil away from her. Gail said to me, "How could you let this happen? I hope you got supervision for this, because you can't help us. You can't quiet the group, and we all want to leave here—it's not safe." This is what she felt and lived with when her mother divorced and married a sadistic bully.

They were right. I had to admit that I had dropped the ball. But what ball did I drop? I could not come up with a way to get Robin to understand what she was so furious and regressed about. I was too thrilled with my own theory, or my pleasure in her recent happiness with her man and new job. I really did like her, as well. I do not think that I was able to hear the craziness in her and in the group's desire to leave or to fire me. Robin was a perfect example of undoing.

This was my unhealthy narcissism running the show. It was fueled by parcels of shame that allowed me to merge with my toxic family and all the fighting that went on there. I was at home with the terrifying rages, ugliness, and disloyalty of my brothers. They did not protect me from the family angst. Instead, I was expected to join my brothers in their hidden shame and rage. When I was 8, my sister was suddenly born, like the new member in the group, and their arrivals instigated major structural and emotional changes in both families. My family dynamics shifted, and I was selected by my mother to be my 8-year-younger sister's parent. Shame and anxiety flooded me, as I was asked to do something I could never do. My toolbox was empty of parenting. I myself needed parenting, and a good lap, which was rarely available. Now I had to *be* the good lap. As William Bendix said in the movie that helped me name my father, *The Hairy Ape*, "What a revolting development."

I did recover from my regression to the Passionate Bad Fit toxic merger, and suddenly knew that I had to remove the paranoid member from the group and then deal with the aftermath, whatever that would be. I needed action, not regression and paralysis. I announced to her and the group that her behavior was too disruptive for her, as well as for all of us, and she would do better seeing someone else. She needed to put her focus on her new love life and new job.

> I will miss you very much. You have accomplished a lot. Your regression was your way of re-merging with your scary mother, and we lost you in the process. This has been inside of you forever and you must have felt safe enough in my lap to let us know directly what you were carrying from your mother as the loyal, faithful, special daughter. We need to get you back, and not you as the scary mother. But you did allow us a look at what you had to go through as a kid, without the protection you needed or a good lap to feel safe in. I thank you for all the good important work and help you have given to others in the group.

The group responded with empathy, warmth, and loving comments about her contributions to them as a favorite member of the group. Some women left later, including Gail, who is still paying me her debt for her group work. She says she feels better, got a job, and seems to feel a little older and maybe more mature. The present group flourishes and we are going to end in about two months. When I retire from running my groups, they will be transferred (if they choose this option) to a colleague after three individual meetings. We will end my connection in two months, after being given a one-year announcement of my retirement. We are all grieving together and laughing at the rough spots, enjoying being close to each other and missing me, as I will miss them.

Chapter 11

Clinical Cases

Glenn

Glenn remained rather indifferent and self-involved, as he felt that he was already in my lap, since I knew his present girlfriend, Jane. He constantly infuriated the group with his preachy sermonettes and paraphrasing of their comments. He was trying to be the therapist but failed each time, and he was always in a quandary as to why this happened to him. One can see that his Passionate Bad Fit with the group was in place rather quickly upon his entry into the group. He was surprisingly misunderstood and impervious to criticism and would seem to be always smiling and pleasant to everyone in the group. For the most part, he acted as if nothing in his behavior in the group was problematic. When I confronted him with this problem, he was surprised, pleasant, and delighted that I took an interest in him. I commented, "It appears to me that you feel there's nothing in this group experience that you find uncomfortable or unpleasant." He agreed and couldn't make much sense out of people's annoyance at times. I asked him if he needed to be in my lap to figure this out; he replied that he didn't really need it at that time, since, except for some problems with Jane, all was going well.

Glenn's seemingly positive transference was a seductive trap to disguise the Omnipotent Child, as well as to suppress the early years of his life and the bad fit with his mother. The therapist's lap to Glenn at this point felt more like the too little, too late lap of his failed father. He didn't experience it as the potential lap of the good-enough mother of infancy. I had to adjust to this shift in order for the lap to be helpful to him and the group. He told us how, when his mother died, he was told that she had taken a lover in another city to have him and did the same thing three years later to have his sister. His father, as far as he knew, never knew that he wasn't their biological father. The father was duped and stayed duped for his own reasons. To be the father in this group, I had to allow myself to be duped by Glenn. I was thinking that I could be his symbiotic mother; instead, I became the devalued father. That didn't negate the offer of the fantasy lap to him, except now the group and I understood why it was refused and could act accordingly.

Glenn filled the group with weekly tales of how much in love he was with Jane, but his stories always had threads of how difficult and demanding Jane was being toward him. He told us how his present wife was giving him a hard time with

DOI: 10.4324/9781032705835-14

their divorce settlement. He was oblivious again to Jane's increasing criticism and demands on him. He would tell us how he would try to please her and to make her smile. He would tell her funny stories, clown around, send her funny gifts, and want to touch her and massage her all the time. He was always calling. He clearly was letting us know how devalued his father must have felt and how powerful women were to him. My dilemma at this time was how to get him to look at the Passionate Bad Fits he was reliving in the group and in his relationship with Jane, in the face of his entrenched Omnipotent Child with its arrogance, loyalty, and passion, soothing recapitulations of earlier Passionate Bad Fits.

I stated over time that Glenn's need to be the most important person in Jane's life and to be the most adored member of the group had led him into terrible traps in relationships. It seemed that to be the most important person in Jane's life was to remain ignorant of any problems and to be devoid of any complaints or to be free of any sense of what he needed other than to be adored.

> If you try to sit in my lap you can let yourself be respected and admired by me and the group, but also you can complain or disagree with me and others in here. You might also find that Christina's unconditional adoration of you hasn't been helpful to you or to her.

Christina didn't like that comment at all, but Glenn remained unmoved at this time. Glenn commented on how Christina got really mad at me and somehow we continued on.

Glenn then talked about Lucien's struggles with me, and how Lucien seemed to have grown through it. He was curious about this for the first time, and actually appeared involved with the group rather than with his own productions and his own smile and physical excitement with himself. I then asked him to tell us what he imagined that first year of life was like for him. He started with how he was conceived and all that must have meant to this mother and father. He was born under the twin drives of deception and denial, and he had lived in that dual identity all his life. He even noticed that at times he would make up characters for himself and take on other people's identities, like the preacher in here, or the meta-therapist in the group. He thought that he must have been the most beautiful child that his mother ever saw. He was a love child, and he still believes in love and the power of being swept away. He imagined that his mother was swept away by a magnificent, handsome man who then became his biological father. He romanticized his beginnings, and he would have many fantasies about him and Jane with another man or woman. These fantasies were intense sexual fantasies that were overpowering and at times overwhelming, almost to the point of being painful. He wanted more and more, and for the sexuality to go on forever. He wanted to be so swept away by the intense feeling of being inside Jane that he would disappear and crawl inside. He excited the group with his tales, and his seduction was powerful, as his mother's was to him. Did I really want this seductive man in my lap? I had to struggle with that until I decided that I could tolerate any sexual feelings that he aroused in me as I tried to hold him. This gave me a clue as to how eroticized his first year of life was. We both needed that experience if we were ever to get to his Omnipotent Child in this treatment experience.

I spoke to Glenn and the group about his need to be in a state of hyper-stimulation. I pointed out to Glenn and the group how he needed the group to intensely focus on him. He needed to be the most important person in the group in order to stay cocooned with his overvaluing mother. He rejected my lap as the lap of his failed father, but he was really trying desperately to stay connected to the earliest intense somatic feelings in both him and his mother at his conception and birth and early years. It allowed the other members of the group to see Glenn in a different way, and therefore not be subject to his seductions and his need to idealize his Omnipotent Child. The group almost always reacts in a highly ambivalently manner as to anyone needing to give up their Omnipotent Child at this phase of the group culture.

These comments did save Glenn from being scapegoated, which for him would have been another highly arousing intimate experience with his Omnipotent Child and the group as the current replacement. Glenn's resistance was slowly worn down, which was greatly aided by the group's increasing awareness of joining him in fostering ties to this Omnipotent Child and to their own. This is a pretty sophisticated group about their own struggles with their own Omnipotent Child. Glenn's resistance was also compromised by my insistence that he try to get close to me, and my interpreting most things he said in the context of his moving closer to or further away from my lap. I also would stop him when he was ready to tell a joke, or to amuse the group with his amorous feats with Jane, or how he could find lots of other women. He eventually had to deal with me and my lap, whether he wanted to or not. All my patients in the group eventually reached this point in their work.

Glenn's lap-sitting and special relationship with me tended to soothe his passionate need for hyper-stimulation and helped him recall with sad affect how his mother disappointed him, how she had other men who shamed him, and how duplicitous she was in her life. He talked of how duplicitous he had also been in his life, with affairs in his first marriage. He was able during this phase to tell the group how his mother gave him breakfast in bed until he was 12 years old, and how shameful exciting, arousing, and humiliating that was, but he was unable to ask her to stop it. He took relief from my stopping him in his over-indulgent behavior in the group. The work with his father, with Jane and other women in his life, awaited all of us, and at some point he may return to the lap to quiet himself as he realizes the tremendous cost to his sense of self the romanticized relationship with his mother was.

Myrna

Myrna saw me in consultation because she was agonizingly trying to decide whether to leave her present therapist and switch to me or someone else. The most apparent and outstanding feature of this session was her ability to agonize so deeply, despairingly, and passionately. I asked her what the issue was with her current therapist, and after explaining it she was able to step back and associate to her lifelong struggle with her mother and father. She found her therapist to be both inadequate and insensitive to her needs (she was charged for a session on a snow day). Her fury was intense, and her ambivalence was equally intense. She also suffered from not being able to decide whether to have a baby. Her history was filled with intense, highly ambivalent, eroticized, engaging, and enraging triangles. Every relationship in her life was highly costly to her self-esteem and to her passion. She clearly had insight and a capacity to do analytic work, but her relationships always interfered with her judgment and her ego capacities. She held on to highly intense, passionate relationships and struggles, which we would be trying to evaluate, explore, and work through in the group. She was highly suspicious of the group but eventually decided to join a twice-weekly group without any individual therapy. She and I were concerned about her neediness. At this point, I pointed out her passion had to do with how much ambivalence and suffering she could endure. I let her know that she would experience me as both her dominating, seductive father and her inadequate, sick, helpless, and angry mother. I encouraged her to let herself feel these passionate feelings toward me and others in the group.

Jesse

When Jesse came into the room for the first time, I felt I was in the presence of the skinny kid in the old Charles Atlas ads who gets sand kicked on him at the beach and if he takes Charles Atlas's course he will be as big and as tough as him. I knew that he needed to be made bigger and tougher, and I had a great deal of compassion and empathy for him because that is the way I saw myself as a child, short and fat and afraid of the world. I got bigger and tougher and so would Jesse. I believed I had a mission with him and had to keep track of those feelings throughout our work. I thought he would get lost in a three-times-a-week group and I was just starting a once-a-week group with combined individual treatment and I thought he would be well suited for that. I guess I didn't want to expose my vulnerability as the sad-sack child to the group and would keep it hidden in the individual sessions. That was not a conscious thought, but in retrospect, I think it was a deciding factor in putting him in the group that I did.

Jesse didn't know how to have fun and never had any, he said sadly. He grew up in a depressed household where his mother lost her beloved first son to leukemia, and Jesse became his replacement. He was given his brother's special ring to wear, and he still wears it. He and his younger sister never really got along and today are miles apart and rarely see each other except at family holidays. Even the holidays were celebrated at the neighbors' house and not his. The neighbors were the main source of pleasure in his life, and he has maintained close ties to the two sisters and brother in that house. They were his surrogate family and were his own family's surrogate for fun and pleasure. It was as if his own family didn't know how to have fun or sustain it over time. His Omnipotent Child very early on encased him in the cave of unhappiness and kept him from venturing out and exploring the dimensions of fun and pleasure.

Jesse felt that his parents never encouraged him to go outside the boundary of his home. He had no friends and was alone all his life. He was quite bright and did well in school but found the social isolation very painful. He didn't seek out any mentors and was dimly aware of his own part in his isolation. He was also aware that he kept waiting for his father to approach him, take charge of the household, and show him how to be a man, which never happened. His father was a very successful accountant and was loved outside the house, but none of that expansiveness was conveyed to him by his father. His father usually worked in the basement or would go on trips to remove himself from his mother's depression and controlling ways. There was no expansiveness allowed, unless it was hidden or secretive. Jesse had always longed to be a doctor, but his attempt at this in medical school away from home was disastrous and painful. He then switched professions and had done quite well, even though he still stayed isolated and quiet at work. His life consisted of going to work, staying alone and competent, and then going home to sleep in his old bedroom. Jesse wasn't athletic and was painfully shy around his peers, especially girls. He had lots of fantasies, but he couldn't act on any of them. He hadn't been with a woman in any way, and at this point in his life felt rather hopeless that this could happen to him. He was terrified of driving a car and didn't until three years before entering treatment. He was afraid of all forms of aggression and assertiveness, both within himself and in the outside world. He had trouble swallowing food and was consistently underweight. He couldn't gain weight, no matter what he ate. He dressed like he didn't expect anyone to notice him or that anyone would expect anything from him.

Jesse's strength was that he was bright, had a great deal of insight, and tried many things, even though he would usually give them up with tremendous feelings of failure, loss, and hopelessness. He used to go to singles events but gave it up after a while, and he went to a social dancing course and painfully left it after he felt that he couldn't keep up with the people there. He regrets that decision profoundly. He never truly settled for a reclusive life, but kept being pulled back there by his past and his present bad fit with his mother and the whole family.

We can assume that, when he was born, his mother was thrilled that he was the replacement for her lost older son, but her enthusiasm for Jesse was not real. His mother, at the same time, was constantly reminded of her loss and her unhappy marriage, so that her grief and joy were intermingled and that left Jesse in the hands of a very ambivalently tortured mother who put her grief into him, as well as her joy for him being someone he wasn't. Jesse didn't know who he was, but he knew who he was supposed to be. This was a paralyzing sense of identity. To be loved meant that he had to be someone else, and to be who he is was to capture all the grief in his mother's life. Therefore fun, pleasure, and excitement for Jesse meant being disloyal to his mother's memories of her son, and to forgo his own identity in his mother's eyes. He was in an impossible situation, and being paralyzed and depressed and staying close to his mother were his only options, since his father was unable and unwilling to bail him out and protect him from this narcissistic bad fit. He preferred that Jesse take his wife's grief and leave him alone to be free to play in the basement. This early bad fit took the juice out of Jesse, and it never returned. He gave up his autonomy to be loved by his mother, not to confront his father, and to keep his father free from his mother's clutches.

Jesse was heroic in his bad fit, as almost all the patients I have worked with are. The insidious heroic aspect of the bad fit is a major ingredient in the creation of the Omnipotent Child. He poignantly and proudly remembered many episodes of family functions when he would be seated with the kids while the adults were inside and he was on the outside. His mother kept him as her lost son both in spirit and design. Anything that took assertiveness and autonomy couldn't be sustained. His wish to be a doctor failed because he couldn't think on his own and create what he needed. He could follow orders but medical school demanded something different and he couldn't do it. His chronic depression and his heroic attachment to the isolation of the Omnipotent Child almost killed him.

He had been in treatment once, but the therapist was not his choice but his mother's, and he lasted for two years but felt he never got better and felt the therapist was an extension of his family and his mother. He felt his autonomy was never encouraged by the therapist. He eventually stopped going about ten years ago. He never picked his own doctor or dentist and always followed orders. He came into treatment with me after being in a car accident that absolutely terrified and immobilized him. He didn't understand his reaction to the accident, where he didn't get physically hurt, except he felt that if he didn't seek help now his life was over. He realized that his only attempt at autonomy, the car, was now over and so was his life. He called an old friend, and she recommended me and he made his first decision to go to a doctor that wasn't recommended by his family.

Jesse would experience his Omnipotent Child as the best friend he had and the only one who could comfort him when he was injured and disappointed and had failed. His Omnipotent Child would reassure him that he was safe in his cave and that no one could reach and hurt him again. This insidious aspect of the Omnipotent Child is the relationship it had with Jesse. It comforted him, but wouldn't let Jesse succeed at what he tried so hard to do, which was to get people in his life other than his family and his internal Omnipotent Child. Day to day, he was frustrated and irritable and depressed enough to try to kill himself, but every day he took comfort in his Omnipotent Child and did not seek treatment on his own and try to break away.

Jesse entered treatment and the group with both apprehension and enthusiasm. He felt this was his last chance to have a normal life and he was going to take it. At first, he wasn't taken very seriously by the others, but since this was a start-up group and he was one of the original members, he had some conferred status on him that he really enjoyed, that he alluded to and then spoke more specifically about later on in his treatment. He soon began to establish himself as the thinker in the group and the analytic one. He was clever, and his insights were truly on target. I felt at times that he was going to be my co-therapist, and later on, since I ran this group by myself, he did in fact assume that role. He began to exhibit his need to be resonant with me in the group. He would sometimes finish my sentences, and I felt that he really understood what I was trying to say to the group and to him. I would

look forward to seeing him in the group and felt more comfortable with his presence in the room. This sense of resonance and the early stages of mutuality were
the first break in the Omnipotent Child position, and the first glance at the potential
good fit that was available to him. He came regularly, and his loyalty to the group
was quite striking. Nothing deterred him from coming to the group. He began to really enjoy the interactions and the verbal battles and insights and most importantly
the awakening in him of a different kind of passion.

Jesse made a connection with an older man who was the most contemptuous,
lonely, angry man I have ever worked with. Howie was deserted early on by his
father, who then committed suicide when Howie was ten years old. Howie quickly
picked up on my special relationship with Jesse as the father-and-son dyad and
began to go after Jesse unrelentingly, without guilt or shame. He attacked him on
all fronts, calling him a weakling, a mama's boy, and attempted to derail all Jesse's
attempts at autonomy and creative action and thinking. Howie hated us and spoke
at length about the rotten and ungenerous son he had and how he hated being a
father to his son. Howie would come into the room ahead of Jesse and take what
he thought was Jesse's chair, which in fact in my other groups is my co-therapist's
chair opposite me. Jesse had assumed the chair before Howie came into the group.
He let it happen for a long time, and through this interaction with Howie, he began to talk of his depression and hopelessness in his life, with an intensity that we
hadn't seen before. I let them both know how difficult it was for either of them to
maintain a healthy lively father–son relationship. I commented that Jesse's return
to his earlier position of hopelessness and despair around Howie's attacks was his
return to his Omnipotent Child position that states, "If I can't have what I need, and
Mother and Father won't let me, and protect me, I will go into my cave and live
there in splendid isolation and without hope." When Jesse saw this as a position he
assumed, he gained new hope and energy from a father rescuing him from Howie
as the aggressive, demeaning, and annihilating mother. He also was able for the
first time to see the aggression in his mother's possessiveness and control. Howie's
presence was the best thing that could have happened to him, and again the beauty
of the group process was, therefore, extremely valuable to Jesse. Confrontation
with Howie opened the path for Jesse to work through these issues.

One day, Jesse raced into the room ahead of Howie and took his old preferred
chair. Howie in his usual way dismissed Jesse's beating him to it and wouldn't
address it with him. With the group's encouragement, Jesse was able to launch
into an attack on Howie, which was a first for him and it shook him up. The group
supported his diatribe against Howie, and the smile on Jesse's face lit up the group
room. They applauded his anger, and everyone felt relieved and peaceful that
Howie was put into his place by Jesse. He reclaimed his seat, and this moment was
a transformational moment in the group for him and for others, which moved him
from the old narcissistic bad fit with his mother to a better fit with me and the group
as the long-awaited rescuing father, and the encouraging, holding, containing, and
resonating family. This transformational moment was the equivalent of his running
home after school, full of aggressive and aroused passions and having a place to

express and experience them with someone, not just by himself—the joy of having his passion resonated with and contained by the most important other in his life. It allowed him to become more energized and vibrant in the group and inside himself, and it allowed for a soothing of his internalized aggression toward himself. As the bad fit began to surrender to the good fit, he began to eat better, feel better, and for the first time began to notice the women in the group, who also for the first time now had to take Jesse more seriously as a man.

His Omnipotent Child was one that existed in a cave that he could retreat into and feel injured and unloved and maltreated, and from which he could fire his mortars in the form of withholding and passive-aggressive behavior. He wasn't going to give anyone what they wanted, even if it killed him. Howie, for Jesse, became, over time, a radar warning for him when he began hearing his voice and having internal conversations with him. He knew then that he was going back into the cave, with his mother inside of him, to stay in her depressed, controlling clutches.

Jesse's passionate, narcissistic bad fit and the resultant Omnipotent Child didn't allow him any fun, pleasure, or sexuality in his life. It kept him with his mother and, while he could vicariously experience an oedipal triumph, the triumph didn't translate into excitement or action. In fantasy, Jesse revealed to the group how his cave contained beautiful things, and how he hoped one day he could have an apartment of his own to put these beautiful things into. He built an imposing cave, with beautiful objects and a lovely bed ready for a woman, but it was sadly still a cave, with no ready entrance to anyone but him and his mother. When Jesse and the group began to underHowied the splendid isolation and its meaning, he began to appreciate how he was holding out on all women to punish them for their controlling ways. They also were punished because they aroused him and wouldn't let him make love to them. His real outrage at his mother was that he worked so hard to stay attached to her, and to be her lost son, but he never won the big prize, going to bed with her. At this time he shared reluctantly his masturbation fantasies of controlling the woman and making her obey all his commands, with potent authority. Being together with someone, even sexually, implied control rather than the pleasures of mutuality.

Concurrently, Jesse discovered Judy, a woman in the group whom he was finding quite attractive. He would sit on the couch with her and gave up his seat opposite me for her, which I encouraged very actively. I would tell him that it was okay that he was moving from me to her, since he still had my support and help to get close to Judy if she wanted that. Judy, who had been burned by men for most of her life, and had been too sexually close to her father, didn't want anything to do with men. Jesse picked a tough one to start with in the group. He wanted to help her, like the group had helped him with Howie, by being the holding, resonating, containing, important person in her life around her painful feelings toward her father and men. She became frightened and rejecting, and experienced his attempts as an incestuous advance. Jesse tolerated the rebuff and reported later that he looked up the company where she worked to get closer to her. Judy expressed her outrage at his invading her privacy, and Jesse for the first time had to look at his own aggression toward the rejecting and arousing woman. It also was a reminder to him and the group how unknowing Jesse had been in making contact with women, and how desperate he had been to be close to a woman, to play and be aroused by her. His joint passions of aggression and sexuality had come out of the cave. Judy brought him out, and he was, for the first time, with good people who could and would want him to live out of the cave. Jesse ultimately appreciated his attempts to be close but told him gently that she cared about him very much, but she just wasn't ready to get that close to anyone, and he wasn't to invade her privacy anymore. He understood and agreed. Now Jesse had to tolerate the anxiety-filled state of the unknown (Agazarian, 1997) giving up the old identity of the Omnipotent Child and forging a new identity without the Omnipotent Child. Jesse was quite relieved when I asked Judy to notice me as the man, which she hadn't done in all her work to date. I told her that, if she kept looking at me and letting herself notice what she thought and felt, she could get over her fear of men.

Shortly thereafter, Jesse got involved with a woman outside the group and had his first sexual encounter. He was thrilled and brought it into the group with great joy and excitement. It was someone he had casually met earlier, who looked him up. He then began to struggle with her reluctance to be more involved with him. What was remarkably clear was his insistence that he wanted more from the woman and from Judy in the group. He was like a starving man who finally found food. He concealed this relationship from his mother for a while, but finally he brought his woman friend over. Shortly thereafter, she dumped him and married, very quickly, someone else. Jesse was devastated, even though he knew she had lots of problems. To everyone's surprise, Jesse went to her wedding uninvited. His assertiveness and power were unmistakably rising and being expressed. I wondered if I wasn't creating a monster. He said that he wasn't going to stay in the cave anymore if he could help it. His only dismay about this impulsive display was having to confront his father's non-resonating, non-empathetic response.

Jesse had another transforming moment with a male member of the group, Kent, who was a big, handsome guy who was married but who used to be a lady's man. He was also a father and had two sons. He would goad Jesse to be more assertive and more masculine, and Jesse didn't know what to do. At one point, they began to tease each other, and he was firing back as good as he was getting. He then wadded a roll of tissues and hurled it at Kent, who was stopped in his tracks, and they both laughed and roared in a play of male bonding and competition that Jesse never had. Another blow to the Omnipotent Child was struck. It was harder for Jesse to stay in the cave anymore. Life was better outside it. He was beginning to understand and experience the joys of mutuality and resonance and fun. He also was paying attention to what the Omnipotent Child was costing him.

Jesse was enjoying life with his new-found aggression, assertiveness, and maleness. He was beginning to carve out his own identity, separate from his mother's, and began noticing that he was quite a man, who could be tough, attractive, and powerful. The women took over and started remaking his appearance, telling him that he needed to change his hairstyle, his eyeglasses, and his choice of clothes.

They dressed him up and changed his persona, and he became a much more attractive and effective-looking man. He no longer would get sand kicked at him at the beach. He hired a clothes stylist and a hair designer, and one day walked into the group and there was a round of applause. He was in a different family and he was in a different fit with himself. The good narcissistic fits were more in place. He went to singles events and began serious dating. Following another serious disappointment with a woman he had been dating, he again returned to the cave for a reattachment with the Omnipotent Child and for some succor. I told him that we were better nurturers than his Omnipotent Child, but to do that he would have to leave his splendid cave and just live with us in this rather nice group room.

This process of rapprochement with a new, better fit, returning periodically after an injury to the cave of the bad fit, lasted for the next two to three years, with increasing autonomy and maturity. He moved out of his family home, bought an apartment, and began to furnish it with the help of one of the neighbor girls that he grew up with. He loved and adored his new home and would bring in pictures and tell everyone about it. Jesse finally found the woman he wanted to marry and, after one year of courtship that seemed rather idyllic, he married her and found himself the stepfather of two teenage sons.

Shortly after the marriage, his wife began to show signs of severe panic attacks, and temper tantrums around not getting her way. She specifically started to separate Jesse from me and the group. He withstood the barrage but was unable to clearly set limits, even though he stayed in the group for another year. He retreated into the cave many times and would withhold from us. We all struggled with his dilemma and would point out the old issues that had resurfaced through this marriage, and how attacking and controlling his wife was. He agreed and was able to see that she had made severe inroads into his place with us in the group. For the first time the group got angry with him, and he retreated further into the cave. He said that he knew that she killed his passion in the group, but being married and being a father was more important. He eventually decided to leave the group, and the usual joyous and exciting departure was not possible, which was truly the saddest point in the group's history. He had come so far, and being stuck in this relationship was so sad for all of us, including Jesse. I knew that the whole group experienced a truly sad moment with Jesse, and the mutuality and resonance of this powerful, enraging, exasperating, painfully passionate moment was another important step in the whole group's maturity. We were able to contain and explore these feelings with him. The group felt unsatisfied in his leaving, but was stronger in their pursuit of the mutual and resonating parts of themselves in the face of the disappointments and the falling off after the excitement pales.

Alex

Alex was a very good-looking, 32-year-old man when we first met in the consultation room. He had been depressed since college, where he drank a great deal, and then never recovered his ability to feel good and have fun. He told me that he had had many years of all kinds of therapy, including group therapy, and nothing had helped him feel undepressed and alive. He had heard that I worked with difficult people who had chronic problems and hoped that I would be able to fix him. I wished I could look like Alex and have all the women love and adore me, yet he couldn't let any woman get close enough to him to even begin to feel that pleasure and/or intensity. I knew that he needed to fall in love and to fight in the group to regain his passion. I asked him if that occurred in his other therapies, and he said rather blandly that it didn't occur and he mostly felt alone and isolated, and when he did say something it was of a whining, complaining nature. I knew that I could offer something better for him in my groups, and I told him so. I told him that I wouldn't allow him to be alone and isolated in the group room and that he would have to deal with me and the others as directly as possible.

Alex grew up in a seemingly ordinary middle-class household where there was no overt trauma, abuse, or neglect that would seem to explain his prolonged depression, which had been immune to a variety of medications and treatments over the last 15 years. His mother was described as a vivacious woman who loved and adored him, and he was the oldest of three children. His father was a salesman who was a frustrated furniture maker, for whom Alex had scorn, contempt, and resentment. He felt his father wasn't helpful enough to him in his early years and was too preoccupied with his own internal dramas and preoccupations. He used to refer to his father as a baboon, and he never felt close to him. Alex was always a good athlete and had many friends. He felt that he was liked as a kid by his peers, and the only thing that he could possibly point to as a traumatic event was the birth of his younger brother when he was 4 years old. He could never say for certain whether this event triggered his mother's moving away from him or if it affected his self-image.

From 5 to 15 he did all the things that a young man does, and he did them well. His schoolwork was good, not exceptional, and he didn't get into trouble or rebel. This, he says, occurred while he was in college, through his heavy drinking and pot smoking. Both his mother and his father needed him to be the best man there could be, and he lived up to that until he got away from his family and went to college. Alex said that he played hard and had to win and be the best there was. He was a star athlete in high school and scored many winning touchdowns. He played basketball and excelled there as well. He never felt happy, but he did all that was expected of him. He dated many girls in high school yet remained rather cool and detached from the experiences. He didn't have fun and felt in retrospect that he was under a lot of pressure to be the best, though he never understood where it came from.

While in his first year of college, a girlfriend of his told him that she was pregnant with his child. He panicked and became obsessed with his badness, and with the awesome responsibility. It turned out that she wasn't pregnant, and this seems to have been a turning point in his internal life. One year later, in his sophomore year, he began drinking heavily and using drugs. This continued for ten years, but then he became afraid that these substances were killing him, and he suddenly stopped using them. At this time, he entered therapy and had been in continual treatment ever since.

Alex's work experience had been spotty, with frequent job changes. His pattern was to work at a job for some time, becoming increasingly doubtful about himself and his work product, and then leave, feeling depressed. He noticed that, whenever he was asked to do something more or to take more responsibility, he would freeze and move into a depressed, obsessed, and self-doubting position, which was his Omnipotent Child. His Omnipotent Child said to the world that it would not tolerate any demands put on him and, if you dared do that, he would become depressed and frustrate you and drive you crazy with anger and hopelessness. His Omnipotent Child would never put a smile on anyone's face again, and no one could make him smile again. Unable to resonate with another's feelings, he left others stuck alone emotionally until they grew enraged enough to leave him.

His relationships with women had been spotty and inconsistent as well. He had dated and had been sexual but could never get too close to a woman. He either broke up the relationship or got too depressed for the woman to stay connected to him. His Omnipotent Child in this arena demanded that the woman both love him and his depression. He could make impossible demands on her, but the rest of the world could not. His sense of mutuality with everyone was terribly distorted. It clearly was a one-way street, where the other person had to put up with his depression, self-doubting, and ambivalence, while he expected that they love him unconditionally. He loved his mother that way, until he began to feel cheated after his siblings were born. He would not resonate with another's passion, and shut them out in the cold, stuck alone with their passionate feelings, saddened and eventually enraged enough that they left him.

When he started this group experience with me, Alex had just changed jobs. He was without a woman and without much real hope for anything better in his life. Where was the narcissistic bad fit and Omnipotent Child in Alex's life? Obviously, from very early on, Alex played a special role in both his mother's and his father's internal life. He was to be the idealized parts of themselves. As the apple of his mother's eye, he was to be the son who fulfilled all her masculine and feminine seductive and sexual wishes and prohibitions. She was a frustrated athlete and skier and wanted a career and a child. She wanted to be famous *and* full with both babies and professional success. She felt that she had married too soon, and wished for a period in her life where she was free to be sexual and irresponsible, and no longer bound to taking care of her father and husband. Her mother died early in her life, and she had to be the caretaker of her angry, unhappy father. She married to get away from her father and got pregnant with Alex within one year. She didn't resent Alex when he was an infant, as he was going to be her ticket to fame, glory, freedom, and excitement. Her ability to be there for Alex, and to resonate with his excitement in the early preverbal phase, was probably very good. He must have felt very attuned and contained by her. The trouble began when he began to separate from her, and she became aware that he no longer was going to be her other self. She got little pleasure from her husband, who was too sad at his own frustrated ambitions. In addition, his father envied Alex his attractiveness and charm and his relationship to his wife.

Alex was clearly the oedipal victor but was the winner long before that. Alex's specialness came crashing down when his younger brother was born when he was three years old. Although he continued to perform and succeed for his mother, she just wasn't as available for him, and the mutuality and resonance was ruptured. He began to resent the responsibility that was thrust on him, just as his mother had with her father. He could never express his resentment to her, since his father was not an ally, and he feared being abandoned like his father was by his mother. His narcissistic bad fits were in the separation–individuation and rapprochement phases, where these personal injuries occurred. One can hypothesize that when Alex's achievements became more his and his alone, there was a reaction in his mother that was not the hoped-for accustomed glowing wonderment.

What about his achievements in the group? How were they responded to? My co-therapist at the time really liked him and I thought that she crossed a boundary with her infatuation and adoration of him. It felt to me like a mother adoring a little boy, who did nothing but look good and make her smile. I, to no one's surprise, reacted to this dynamic. I called it out. And spoke many times to her, and we wound up agreeing that we would disagree on her work with Alex. I was supposed to be the adored one, so I had to keep watch closely on my own competitiveness, being the fourth boy in a family of five children.

While this was happening, Alex fell in love with Helen, a member of the group, and they plotted seeing each other outside of group, or running away and getting married. They both took it hard when I said no to these plans, and Alex got angry in the group for the first time. He was no longer the cute, adorable little boy. He was an angry, mean, powerful, and scary guy, to me and the group. He no longer was living in the toxic merger with his adoring, non-demanding mother.

I have noticed that some patients create difficult positions for themselves so that they can realize the toxic merger and start escaping from it. Alex stepped into the first reflections of the Passionate Good Fit, and began to feel all the dilemmas of that space. He got confused, disoriented at times, and said he was unsure of who he was, unsure that he liked himself that way. He felt more alone, yet healthier than he had ever felt. He could not make sense of his emotions, like his anger and his willfulness.

He reported an old dream of nearly scoring a touchdown for his high-school team but deliberately falling down just before the goal line. He cried as he began to see that this was how he ran his life. Almost the best, but really just an addict and a drunk—but always cute.

He terminated with us in a healthy manner and began to enjoy his newfound freedom to work, love, and be happy. He changed his job and grieved over his unrequited love for Helen, but thought that he could feel both love and gratitude, as well as the pleasure of having worked so hard in therapy and accomplished so much. He thanked us sincerely, and we were all able to smile with a job well done.

Marsha

Marsha entered my training group because she thought that I could enliven her life and stir up her energy and excitement. She had been in one of my AGPA Institutes and liked her experience there and how I worked with the Omnipotent Child. Now she believes she is living in hers but cannot stop herself, and hopes that working with me would enable her to come more to life. She also knows some people who were going to join my newly formed therapist training group that meets twice yearly for two weekends per year. That group is now in its 28th year and is facing its complicated and sad ending.

Marsha is a 50-year-old married mother of a married son, living in the NorHollyst Corridor. She grew up in an eastern Slavic country that was always at war. She remembers the shelling, and always had to be wary of going outside, or even being curious about anything that would make her leave her closed-in home. Everyone was terrified, and her mother would tell her daily to try to avoid being killed by the bullets. Her early trauma was painful to hear, but she told it with an indifference that was striking. It was as if this is part of her life, and that is the reality she lives in. She cannot feel the rage, the despair, or the fear of her childhood, but has deadened herself in order to go on living, have a career, raise her son, and be unhappily married. She has tried different forms of therapy before, to no avail. Her indifference covers her desperation to live again, but there was something she saw and felt about my zest for life that let her try to live, and she decided to give me a try. She entered the biannual training group.

To no one's surprise, she is quiet, proper, listening to the others, but rather nonresponsive to the early symbiotic mother. She is courteous and the group loves her, as she sort of becomes the group mascot. I did not exist for her at the beginning. I was hurt and then realized that she wanted me to feel how killed off she was in her early and present life. Now we can start talking, as we talk about what it is like to be killed off, to fear death every day, and to have no one really understand it. We discuss how to be alone with it. She rarely talks to anyone about her early life. The group senses her fragility, and the courage it takes to be with us. They are very careful not to jar her, except for Janny. He could not care less. He is a bully, who came from that area of the world that Marsha had come from. He is a very unhappy camper and feels that the only thing he can own is not letting anyone in and surrendering. He too shares stories of the war that he has endured. So they are face to face—the bully and the victim. But both were victims of early traumatic injuries, which led to highly punishing Passionate Bad Fits. Neither can enjoy intimacy, though they both try so hard. Janny engages the group and me, but he makes it quite known that he has really powerful limits to intimacy. "So what are you going to do with me?" I ask him and her too, at different times in the group work.

At this point in the work, I make a conscious decision to try to reach Marsha instead of Janny. I think she is more reachable. As her deadness increases in the room, even with my prodding her about her relationship with me as the symbiotic mother, I say that her Omnipotent Child is how she can thrive in her sadness and still live her life. I say that was her construction to deal with the terrible injuries to her safety and to her narcissism. Her narcissism was embedded in the heroic bad fit of how magnificently she could live, while dead, and not notice her losses and the heavy price she paid, not having love, intimacy, and warmth in her life. I say,

> You've built a monument to your deadness, and we should therefore honor that, as you honor it. We should, with your help, including Janny, build you the most wonderful, most magnificent coffin there ever was, and that will be your place when you meet with us. You will have a great deal of say as to the insides of the coffin, the material, anything you want in it, and how comfortable it should be for you.

She smiles and asks whether we are serious about this coffin stuff. I and the group say yes, absolutely. A new and different Marsha arrives at the next session—she is a different person. She speaks, cries, and says that no one had ever taken her seriously about living in death every day. Janny even ventures a comment of support for her newness. (This group only meets for a weekend every six months.)

The Process of Building the Coffin

It takes us two full weekends, six months apart, to build the coffin. We start with the composition of the material of the coffin itself. The group laughs and then speaks of their own shame in living in their Passionate Bid Fit, which cannot be put in a coffin. It is too diverse, not as specific as Marsha's is, they say.

They try to speak of their conflicted relationships. One member says she has been living in a constant war with her mother for years, with no solution possible. It used to occur when her mother tried to brush her long hair and she never felt taken care of; instead she felt like her mother wanted to hurt her. I have to continually get the group back to the construction of the coffin. They alternate with excitement and then resistance and indifference to the building of the coffin. I let the group know that their envy, competition, and awareness of the death they have been living in has increased their resistance to helping build the coffin. "You are nuts," they say. I say, "No one has done this, since I have been around. Are you so sure you are honoring her Omnipotent Child or your own?" Marsha sometimes has to bring the group back to the construction process. She is in it, and wants a strong wood coffin that will never be destroyed, that would last forever. She enjoys picking out different woods, letting herself slowly come back to life. The group sometimes expresses their admiration and puzzlement at her mood change. She is alive now, and who is she to us now? What will Janny do? Who will he silence, or bully? Marsha wants someone special to construct the coffin, someone who really knows his carpentry. "I want it to be perfect," she says. "I am delighted," she says, after telling us that the worker did the right job. She is happy with it and then wants to climb in, just see if it fits. We are seeing the neutralization of the unhealthy narcissism, slowly shifting to a healthier narcissism, as she builds her coffin with gusto, relish, and excitement. The coffin lets her cross the Rubicon.

Marsha exclaims, "It fits!" Some of the others want to join her in the coffin, and shamefully admit that they are just a little bit jealous and envious. But do they want to be dead to get this special caring? She begins to go from a mascot to a middle-aged, attractive woman now. Her smile is flirtatious and charming. She wants to fill the coffin with special materials to comfort her on her long rest. She chooses, with a great deal of excitement, a red silk, lush, soft, and elegant robe and cover to reside in and luxuriate in. The coffin becomes a boudoir for her and the group. Lots of discussion ensues about the group's sexuality, and their reluctance to talk about it. They are trying to go beyond their shame, as they see Marsha go beyond hers as she lies in the coffin. She feels all dressed up now, like she is at a debutante coming-out party. The change is incredible, the excitement is intoxicating, and we are all caught up in it. Her death would not let her vibrancy and sexuality come to the fore—that would be too disloyal. She says that her new-found liveness can tolerate being disloyal. Memories of earlier excitements fill the room. Janny even talks about pleasant moments with his former wife and children.

Marsha now struggles with how new she can let herself be. She begins to tell stories of the horrific past that she survived. She really begins to notice me and talks about how she had to push me away; she apologizes for her behavior. She wants to know who owns the coffin. Can she keep it and take it home with her? I let her know that it is always hers, she owns it, and the attachments she makes here are hers to keep. I say,

> Your new-found Passionate Good Fit is yours to own as well. No one is going to strong-arm you and take it away, but our work now will be to help you keep your new-found identity and attachments, and help you to understand when you want to undo it.

She gets into the coffin regularly for at least two to three years of our meetings. She then announces that she no longer needs to be in the beautiful coffin that saved her life.

At this point, Marsha adds individual therapy, where she continues the exploration of her deadness. From the coffin, she is able to make the connections of her past fears and traumas, and shame, that staying alive was tantamount to a devastating betrayal of the family's need to live in death. Her disloyalty put her in a terrible dilemma. Which way will her conflict be solved? Which way will her narcissism go? Her unhealthy narcissism cannot allow her to be disloyal, so she holds on to her Bad Fit even tighter and more heroically. Through the symbolic coffin, we are taking her Passionate Bad Fit to its extreme. (A gestalt therapist might have built her an actual coffin, but not in the same theoretical context of my work.) She is able to begin a slow but steady process of neutralizing the unhealthy narcissism. Janny's presence in the group also enables her to confront the bully, the dangerous war machine, and survive. She sees his vulnerability as well, and they are both, over time, able to have empathy and sadness for each other's life.

Marsha continues to grow, stays for a long time in the group, and is able, with the group's help, to see that she is trying to undo her new Passionate Good Fit. She begins to see that leaving the group felt as if she would be disloyal to us and to the coffin. She struggles with whether she will allow herself to cross the Rubicon and live in the Passionate Good Fit. This is a crucial part of the work in the group—to acknowledge that you are and will be disloyal to the old Passionate Bad Fit, and survive and deal with the siren call to undo the gains and stay loyal. This is the hardest and longest part of her therapy and, thankfully, it is successful. We have to get her to recognize that she no longer needs the group, and she should leave and go to Europe with her new-found husband and with her new-found life and loves.

Debra

These are the last few sessions with Debra, both in the group and in the individual work. She begins to understand the deadly triangle that she was stuck in very early in her life. Only now can she understand it, work with it, and feel the dilemma.

She would never allow us to do any work on her feelings toward her mother. She needed to protect her at all costs, even giving up enjoying her femaleness, her love life, her potential children, and her sexual and feminine body. Her body, as in most Passionate Bad Fits, became her enemy for most of her life. She could be sexual, but never with a man she could have. How she loved her mother! She never said how Mother loved her.

In the group she took more risks: to speak out, to become the leader of the group, and to be highly regarded for her participation. As she let herself thrive in the group, and take ownership of her gifts, she began to allow herself to talk about her mother. Both her parents died about two years ago, so the rest of the story happens after their deaths.

In the individual work, which was once a week (as was group), she began to appreciate me as a trusting man who she could adore and learn from. Her relationship with her father was fraught with high tension and mutual hurting, which left her unprotected from his rages and ugly comments about her. Her mother never protected her from Daddy, she would say, but Debra always knew that Mother would die for her if she was in danger. She never could solve the internal confusion of feelings toward her beloved mother, but now she was able to contemplate that dilemma. She could never let herself solve it; instead, she would feel shame that she did not protect Mother enough. She also began to realize that carrying extra weight was symbolic of carrying her mother's shame. She was protecting Mother from the shame of using Debra to escape Father's rages. Debra subconsciously was put into a deadly triangle, where Mother gave her to Father, then acted fragile so she could get Debra to care for her and never get angry with her. Debra tended to play this out in various high-profile jobs. She never thought that she got the respect in those jobs that others did. She tended to leave jobs when she hit her peak, because she thought she couldn't go further and get the top job. A new job came up for her to evaluate, and we worked together forecasting her Passionate Bad Fit choices, and how she could not let herself enjoy her successes. She could not let herself enjoy and appreciate the great job she was doing at this place. She, in fact, had caught the brass ring, but her Passionate Bad Fit would not let her truly appreciate how successful she was. Her success got lost in the agony and shame of wanting more, being ultimately denied that specific reward, and being stuck with shame, angst, low energy, and feelings of depression and loss.

About two months ago, she got a dog from the pound that was five years old and was reared in the house of a very disturbed woman who at times would abandon him. Debra had never had a dog; she has had two cats for years. She named the dog Moose, because Mother had a connection to that name. Her mother would tell her that, if she ran into a moose, Mother would attack and kill the moose to protect Debra, the little girl. Getting the dog was a big risk, to help her to move from the Passionate Bad Fit to the Passionate Good Fit, and to satisfy her need for change. She was also redoing her house and suddenly realized that the renovations were going to be for her, not for the next family that bought the house.

I kept supporting her growth, her risks, her curiosity, her new-found dreams, enjoying new-found sexual fantasies, and liking her insides more than ever. She was smiling more, looking more attractive, and exuding warmth and trust in our interactions, as she had in the group. She was ready to tackle the mother issue. This was heralded by her asking a more hidden member of the group, "Do you love me? Do you love us?"—the long-awaited voice of the infant after the wordless phase of her development. She asked the unspoken question that most children would have liked to ask and could not.

I believe that my work was validated by the questions, and by the way Debra and others have the ability and desire to put more words to that wordless body experience. This plaintive question touched us all. I felt so moved that I was close to tears. It felt to me that my theory and techniques were bearing fruit.

At the same time, she was clearly becoming, to me and the group, a more attractive woman, with whom we all enjoyed working. She let go of position changes at work that would have landed her in the Passionate Bad Fit, and began to joke and laugh with me about her actions. She was finally developing an observing ego and could now laugh at her exploits rather than use them to keep shame as the organizer of her internal life. In the group, she would ask hard questions and make powerful comments about herself and others' behavior in the group and outside.

In a recent individual session, she again brought up her concerns about Moose with her two cats. The cats and Moose are still walled off from each other, on the advice of a trainer. Her friend, who loves dogs, put her into conflict when he suggested that she was not helping Moose and letting the dog grow. He implied that she should not have gotten Moose, and only got him for own pleasure, but was not understanding of his needs. She was quite hurt by his comments, but they struck home with her. She believed that she made Moose hostage to her house, and yet was also a parent to him. She regretted the decision to get him, even though the dog is not complaining and is in fact thriving every day. She takes him to nurseries and walks him on the leash for company with other dogs. Clearly, she is not an abusive, neglectful, or selfish parent to Moose. Her clear role as the caring respectful parent could not contain the pull of the Passionate Bad Fit, and a classic undoing began inside of her. This time she was able to stop the slide, by observing it and noticing the signs inside her: lack of energy, sleeplessness, and a feeling that she just isn't good enough.

We then described her slide into the Passionate Bad Fit. Her friend's comments stirred up a lot of shame. This shame then activated the Passionate Bad Fit and all the unhealthy narcissism and grandiosity that went with it. She then re-merged with the deadly triangle from her youth. This is the crucial factor in accumulating shame, which drives and organizes the Passionate Bad Fit. So we can ask, who is she merged with? Her old family triangle, or me and the group as her new family? The backsliding also kills or corrupts any gains that may have been made. Shame is the crucial component in her backsliding, but the backsliding did let us use this time to investigate how trapped and stuck she was in her family, fighting and hating Father. I pointed out, "I never heard you say that Mother said how much she loves you. You only said it about your feelings toward her." Once I had pointed out the power of shame, she tried to recount all the ways that she was not the parent she said she was. She was not going to buy what I was selling.

I helped her recognize the dilemma she had had all her life about Mother. She always thought that her mother protected her from the dangerous world but did not protect her from Father's anger and negative feelings about women. Mother gave her to Father so she could be free of his rages and live more safely. She was shocked when she realized that her mother used her too, and that finally helped explain why Mother never asked her about her normal life as a teenager or as an adult woman. She never asked, where are the boys? Do you want a family? What are your goals in life? Debra regretfully acknowledged that she was held hostage, as she thought she was doing to her dog. She became aware of the conflict with her mother. She thought her mother protected her from the world. At the same time, she was being used in the triangle by both Mother and Father. She finally let herself express anger toward Mother, which she never did before. She was relieved. Now she understood why she was able to ask those questions in group: "Do you love me? Do you love us?"

The group has now been graduating, as I near my planned retirement from group work after giving a one-year notice of my intent. Now they are talking openly about love. Is it connected to having to keep pleasing the other? Is it a burden that ties us down? How do we live with the fact that none of us was ever loved the way we needed to be? Their combined answer was

We need to develop enough good radar and use the work we have done in here, to be disloyal to the toxic mergers in which we all grew up. We have to try to hold on to Dr. Aledort's healthy narcissism and the joy he gets from it. We must continue to live in the Passionate Good Fit and no longer carry anyone else's shame. We have to be ever aware of the pull to undo the new connections, and remain loyal to our old toxic mergers. We are ready to end.

And so was I, with a big smile on my face, filled with tears of joy, happiness, success, and a profound pleasure and honor to have worked with this group for so many years.

Laura

Here's a case that illustrates the Omnipotent Child and the Passionate Bad Fit. Laura, a 45-year-old married woman, entered the group because of life-long depression and inability to create and sustain good opportunities for herself. She is presently unemployed; her husband is a high-school teacher. During the evaluation, she was able to talk about how she sabotaged herself, but previous therapy did not change that. She looked like a lost, anxiety-ridden girl searching but never expecting a good lap.

When she enters the ongoing group, she is wrapped in a hoodie and sits in a corner close to me. She says nothing. I say, "The group will learn as they watch you enter the group. In the meantime, you and I can talk, and you don't have to respond, unless you want to." She reminded me of Bartleby, the Melville character who spent his adult life saying, "I prefer not to." I start the interaction by commenting on her hoodie.

STU: You look like you're making a lap for yourself. When you're ready, my lap is always present. You're scared, I get that. You cannot trust us, like we cannot trust you yet. You smiled. I think I hit pay dirt.

LAURA: I have nothing to say.

STU: That's fine, because your body is telling us so much in the only way it can, which is not words. Your hoodie is great. You want to be enveloped, but you're terrified that you will not be fed well again. You do look like you do not eat well.

LAURA: I don't eat well and I'm not sure I like you. You act like a know-it-all.

STU: I do want to get to know as much of you as you will permit. We could grow together, over time. You just told me three very important things that are a central part of telling your story. You can relax. We'll sit in silence.

We gaze at each other, and the group gazes at both of us, quietly but intensely listening, remembering their own entrance to the room, which they share later on. The women in the group want to hold her, cry with her, and tell her it will work out. "You have come to the right group." I interrupt them and tell them, "Your empathy is clear and beautiful, but she needs to tell her story with and to me. How are we going to know which trauma and misattunements hurt her the most? And began to form the beginnings of the Omnipotent Child through her body?" It feels like a group of somatic feelings, like her intermittent hunger, helplessness, sorrow, and rage, fuel the first laying down of the Omnipotent Child. These somatically induced neuronal dendrites begin to organize and lay down a network in parts of the right cerebral hemisphere.

This cluster of somatically driven feeling-states get imbedded in new neuronal circuits and begin to make themselves known, especially if there are repeated misattunements that occur around feeding and holding with the all-knowing mother. This constellation is most likely situated in the body ego, and the Omnipotent Child is the reservoir of all these feeling states of the preverbal phase of life. It is fueled by the primitive narcissism of the body ego, which lends it power, and the need to define oneself in this period of growth. The primitive identity that is formed becomes a central staple of the child's identity. Freedman (1989) postulates that the following conflict-free psychobiological needs form the basis for the infant's core identity: curiosity; excitement; sense of self; self-differentiation; the self's view of the body as either enemy or ally; and the sense of self as either good, calm, and contained, or disorganized, disruptive, and inconstant. These healthy core identities of the infant are put at risk when the body ego experiences a failure in the relationship between the mother and the infant. When these moments of failure are filled with high intensity, the healthy core identities get corrupted, and the passion of these moments takes over and becomes the source of the child's core identity, foreshadowing the relationships with others and with the self. This is the beginning of the Passionate Bad Fit (Aledort, 2002).

STU: How are you feeling, sitting with all of us? I really want you to see me as the most important person in the group. I've been through this period of work with all the group members you see here today. It'll give us a chance to put into words feelings that are now stuck in your body about those first years of your life. We have plenty of time.

LAURA: I really don't like you, and that feeling is growing stronger every time you talk. You're stingy with all of us. You act as if you know me more than I do, and who in hell said you were the most important person in the group?

STU: I notice that you took the hoodie off your face, and now we can see each other better. I'm presumptuous. I do feel powerful, but also feel anxious about you being my new infant. How was your mother stingy to you?

LAURA: I'm not talking to you, or to anyone else. I didn't want to be your infant. That's why I never had a child, and never will.

STU: That must hurt deep inside of you, that the past without words could have such a powerful influence on how you decide to run your life. It might be helpful if we began to understand that intimate time in your life.

LAURA: I take pride in not being happy, in not doing what's expected of me, and driving people crazy.

STU: Could you drive me crazy and win the battle? Of course. But I'm a worthy opponent, as you'll hear from the other members. I endure, I keep working, I keep searching for your truth and for your story to be put into words.

BUDDY   [another group member]: Come on, Laura, stop fighting and come join us as infants who are learning about intimacy and our power and our helplessness. Come join us.

This period of exploration of the mother–child dyad takes about one year for the elucidation of the Omnipotent Child and the subsequent Passionate Bad Fit in a form that can be understood by the patient. The rest of this time is spent with further clarification of all the bad fits in the feeding and holding in the dyad. Laura is trying to notice that these early experiences shaped and corrupted her healthy core identities. Instead, she became distrustful, hated her body, and kept trying to live in the helplessness, rage, and longing of infanthood. She began to smile, she began to talk, and she joined the group to become one of the more impassioned defenders of the group process, while still being very suspicious of me and my motives. The Bad Fit always needs a place to sit and exert its influence. It has become the most important part of the identity and it is incredibly difficult to be disloyal to it. Heroism is needed to separate from this identity. Most people do not, even with different models of therapy.

Thumbelina

Frances is referred to me through a friend of hers I work with, who has done very well in putting her life back together again. Frances is depressed, she says, has trouble sleeping, and does not seem interested in having sex with her husband. She cannot figure that out, since she feels she loves him, but she won't let herself get too excited. She has a demanding job that she is quite good at. She loves to get things accomplished and cleaned up. She does not like messes. She thinks that sex is messy and tries to avoid it, on those grounds. She makes eye contact with me easily, has a pleasant smile, and is clearly the businesswoman in these first interviews. She sees herself as a social animal, and so thinks that my group might help her. I ask her, "With what do you need help?" "With everything," she says with a smile. She tells me that she has had previous therapy, but not group. She is willing to try, since at times she feels desperate and cannot figure out why she would feel this way. She has everything. It is a mess that the other therapies did not fix properly. She is not afraid to lose her husband; she feels her marriage is solid and on the right track. She has not had any affairs and she believes that she suffers from low libido, unlike her high energy when it comes to work.

My first impression is that she will do very well in the group and become one of the leaders. I am looking forward to struggles with her around my passion and her lack of it. I think she will try to help the others in the group, before she can get serious about her own condition. She will struggle with us about loosening up, as opposed to her very closed-in and almost camouflaged appearance. I think about how tightly she wears her hair, and what would she be and who would she be if she let her hair down? I love my thoughts about Frances. Was I already trying to fill myself up, because maybe Frances might drain me, and I had to fill myself, rather depend on her? *Great questions*, I think to myself.

She enters the room, quiet, self-composed, looking like she has everything under her control. No messes showing. She does not display a great deal of anxiety upon entering the treatment. She does not appear to me to be depressed. The original back-and-forth around her being a newborn (a new group member) is met with quiet determination to get it right, and try to answer and dialogue with me. I picture a little girl who never got dirty, who always smiled to make her mother smile, and who went through life trying to keep smiling, but finally could no longer do it. She looks as if she could explode with tears and rage, and tremendous fear. She becomes a staple for the group. We all know that Frances would be there, composed and making no demands of us. She becomes a model for the group of the perfect daughter. They rarely make demands on her either. Everyone is content, except me. I have to know who she is behind this veil of propriety and calmness. After one year in the group, she becomes more silent and rarely speaks. The group does not encourage it, but they do not demand that she speak to them and be more alive in the group. She is able to quietly, without rancor, push these questions and demands to the side, including mine. I become concerned, intensely frustrated by her charming no. She reminds me of Bartleby, by Melville—"I would prefer not to speak." We have no idea of her relations at home, with her husband, her mother and father, and her peers. When we start asking these questions, at my insistence, she usually gives one-word answers. She appears to listen to the others in the group but rarely engages them fully. I begin sessions now, by asking Frances if she has anything to say today or report on anything that she might have noticed either at work, or with her husband or her parents. I assume this was the aloneness of the early years of her life.

In my office, there is a glass table that holds crystalline figures that patients have given me as they left treatment. There is also a *papier maché* duck with a plant in its middle. At various times, patients in different groups would comment on the figures and wonder who gave them to me and how I felt about them. There was always a lot of fantasy about the figures, and each group had a different relationship to these figurines.

Frances always sits next to the table and I see her scrutinizing the figures, smiling sometimes, but usually silent as to what is in her thoughts. I ask her if they stir up fantasies or dreams in her mind, and tell her that she feels to me that she is afraid of what is inside of her. She denies any memory of a traumatic episode in her childhood. She never reports dreams. When asked how she is feeling that day, she usually says that she is OK. She never reports any moments of high anxiety, depressions, or obsessive thinking. She just gets through the days, in neutral gear. She does want to feel more, she says, and recognizes how empty she is, and how lonely. Life never really warms her up. She has friends of long standing, who put up with her quietness and reserve. She cannot recall any impulsive feelings or action in her childhood or her adult life. Her marriage is sober, conventional, without a lot of passion for either of them. They have no kids, and she says that is OK with her. This material about her passionless life slowly emerges over time, and she seems to feel closer to another woman in the group. They talk and nod heads in agreement about what others may have felt. The group again does not express any rage, frustration, or annoyance with her silence. "Frances is Frances," they say in agreement. At no time, do I or the group see her silence as resistance or hidden aggression. She just has nothing to say, which reflects her passionless life of the pre-oedipal time.

I assume that her first year of life was one of not making a mess for her mother. I assume she did not scream too loudly, was compliant with mother's needs, was the good child, and made no demands on her mother. She cannot remember, but this is what we piece together of her earlier life. She tends to assume we are correct. Her speculations about her mother are that she did not bargain for children, wanted to be a lawyer, did not like children, avoided kids' parties, and led a small life. She rarely saw her parents feel strongly about anything. Impulsive behavior was almost absent in the family. Frances had kid friends, played a lot, and tended to avoid being home, but she did not adopt another surrogate family to satisfy her needs. Her joy and pleasure were corrupted by her parents, even though we have no evidence for that at this time in our work.

After about two years of therapy, in which she is 75% silent but with us as a listening, connected person who does respond to others in the group and is well liked by them, she suddenly raises her hand and says, "I have something to say. The Duck ate the Mouse." We are all flabbergasted by the comment, as well as by her delivery. She takes over the room on the table, the silent one, awakened. This event takes place after the nightly cleaning crew moved the mouse to a bookcase in a corner of the group room. The mouse was not on the table. She says how afraid she is, how anxious she has become, and how this makes no sense to her.

> But what happened to the little mouse? I love that little mouse. No, I do not name her, but she is a little girl. She was my silent friend during all these years of silence. I don't know why, I tried my best to figure it out by myself, because I was too ashamed to tell you about my attraction and attention and companionship to the little mouse.

The group has many associations to Frances's story, about their connection with figurines on the table, and then to the pictures in my office, then to who are those girls in those pictures? Curiosity, intrigue, and unconscious questions flood the group. Frances now joins and is a highly active member in the group. We all smile a lot and are all happy with her participation at this time. I feel vindicated in not pushing her as I thought I should. She was the sleeping child in my lap, in my theoretical posture. She needed to feel safe enough to talk, to be, to exist. I did not know that the mouse was in her lap. We all create our own lap but do not know how to use it or feel entitled to have it. She does. She is going to make this room her place of safety, any way she can, and she does. One month later, she reports her first dream. She is pregnant and delivers a large sac that has a dead little girl baby in it. She cries when telling us this dream and is puzzled by it. We talk about who and what the dead baby represents. She says, "It must be me, but what part of me?" I tell her,

> Maybe it is your aliveness. Look how alive you are now, and how you, in your own way, played as if you were dead in here, or was killed off. You could only relate to an un-live figure, your mouse. Even the mouse comes to harm, when the duck eats it.

She looks around and spots the mouse on the bookshelf, and smiles as if she has found the love of her life. Frances begins to see how the duck was her mother who killed off her excitement. She feels that her role was to make mother smile, an impossible task at which she failed. Her success came when she carried her mother's shame all her life. Then she was heroic, proud, felt alive but knew that she could only belong to mother and her assigned task. She is totally entrenched in living in the Passionate Bad Fit. Her Omnipotent Child is how magnificently she can carry Mother's shame and still make a living, still get married, still be respected by her peers, but dead to the rest of her emotional life, pleasure, excitement, and sexuality. Her narcissism is embedded in the heroic Bad Fit, and therefore not available to her everyday life. She lives in a state of unhealthy narcissism, like how long she could go without talking to us. Heroic and magnificent! How long can she go on carrying her mother's shame of being a negligent mother to her? She tries to invigorate herself in many ways but always feels that she can never let herself be excited about anything. That would be treasonous and disloyal. She has lived in her Passionate Bad Fit all her life, until now. She could feel her excitement but was terrified that she would or someone or something would destroy it, like the duck and the mouse.

This resonates with the group as they commiserate with each other about their loss of excitement, of the position of having to take care of the parent versus being taken care of. They talk about the loneliness in their lives, when they have been cut off from their dreams, exciting fantasies, sexuality, and enjoyment, except on rare occasions. It is hard for patients to bring in dreams, since it requires a sense of internal safety and trust of your unconscious as well as basic trust in your integrity and your specialness and uniqueness. I have come to believe that every patient needs an unconscious moment in their lives or in the therapy, to be able to go deeper and begin to live with the mysteries of the unconscious.

In the midst of the excitement in the group, about discovering sexuality, asking the questions of early childhood, "show me yours and I will show you mine," Frances comes forward with another blockbuster dream. She dreams that as she is resting on a couch at home, there appears a dancing figure, in a red ballet outfit, twirling on the table and looking so real. "I was entranced by her twirling, her smile on her face and her little ballet outfit." Who is she? She associates to her early years, when she did take ballet, and how the lessons were stopped by her mother for reasons that never made sense to Frances. She thinks that the figure was no bigger than her thumb. We all say, "It must be Thumbelina." But who is Thumbelina to her? We all associate to many different things, like her excitement, how she has been twirling in her Bad Fit, and how she would like to twirl like her. I suggest that it might be her clitoris. That stops the group for a moment, but then Frances says that it would be the right size.

> I haven't touched or masturbated myself for ages. Do you think that it means that I might be ready to feel and touch myself and get reunited with my body, as

I used to like myself when I was younger? But it was a dirty, shameful experience that eventually went the way of all the other excitements in my life and body.

"I am ready," Thumbelina calls. Frances continues in the group for another year and grapples with siren calls to return to the loyal Passionate Bad Fit and take comfort in never being disloyal. But now she has a real lap that is filled with healthy narcissism and excitement. She is the new Frances, and we all love her for the changes that occur in the group work. I smile because it confirms again for me that my theory has merit and works appropriately, really helps make character change and maintain it. Years later, she writes to say, "I and my husband are alive and well, there is a child now, a little boy, and we think of you often. Thank you so much."

Chapter 12

The Risks in the Work

Patients have to take risks in the group to move from the Passionate Bad Fit to the Passionate Good Fit. Throughout the work, I stress at various times their need to take those risks. The biggest risk that *I* have to take is acknowledging my own shame at my mistakes: not paying enough attention; thinking more about myself than about the group; forgetting a patient's name. I even feel slightly skittish when I know that my lifelong dream of being a great actor or radio star spills over and I get carried away with my interpretations and my own magnificence.

I deal with the shame of exposing my narcissism with humor, and with a little boy's facial expressions. I really can laugh at my own foibles, and I think that it softens me as I process the hard work of the unconscious material, the theory, and the clinical interventions. I am "on" a lot of the time, and I really enjoy the spotlight, which led me to posit that I am the most important person in the room. It fits me and fits with the theory, which is no surprise because every theory has parts of us incorporated within.

Exposing my theory and my practice to the AGPA membership felt like a huge risk, and yet I believed I had to do it to find out if I was right and why. As time went by, AGPA was extremely helpful in modifying my practice and my theory, and it allowed me to enjoy my narcissism in the fruitful endeavor of discovery and creation. I knew I had to create something but was never sure what it was and how it would get expressed.

Through my AGPA experience, I realized that my patients had to take big risks in their lives in order to harness healthy narcissism, rather than stay in the unhealthy, shame-driven narcissism. This part of the work developed later, as I kept noticing patients' need to undo the gains they had made, and their reluctance to be disloyal to the earliest toxic mergers of infancy and childhood.

My own risk-taking allowed me to be disloyal to my parents' smallness and to my brother's unhealthy narcissism. I had followed him professionally, because I thought that I too could be a good doctor, just not like him. In being disloyal, I fought with him a great deal: we struggled over a common girlfriend, we teased each other endlessly, and we finally realized there was little room for us both, and very little to like about each other. We are both successful doctors, and both widowed now, but we still rarely communicate with each other.

DOI: 10.4324/9781032705835-15

If you do not take a risk in the group, you will not be able to move away from the Passionate Bad Fit. Frances finally risked sharing with us her terrifying fantasy that the duck ate the mouse. Bruce was able to fall in love in the group, and express his rage at Ken, the bad father. Alex was able to stand up to his tormentor in the group, which led to his setting firm limits on his wife's behavior. A long-standing patient of mine, whom we loved and admired for our work together, was able to find a different therapist for his family, to help him with his son's acting out. He struggled with this act of disloyalty to me and to our work. He imagined I would be furious with him, and see him only as a sad, bad little boy, until I told him that I was delighted that he had found someone who could help him, when I was too limited.

A quiet woman who wanted to live in the shadows of the group was able to leave her sadistic husband after twenty years of abuse. She adored me and my power. She was able to get involved with a very difficult man, who was very wrapped up in himself. She would talk about her struggle to decide whether she should leave him or stay. She got stuck in that internal dynamic with herself and with the group. The one day she suddenly told us that she had bought a magnificent house in her ideal vacation spot. This opened the door to all of us helping her confront the issue of whether, in this remote location, he would be able to take care of her, if she needed. By buying the house, she had made herself confront her painful childhood, in which she had to take care of herself as her parents acted like little children. She had to be the parent, and never had looked at how lonely she felt without her parents being available to her. All internal systems became alive, as she got out of the shadows and worked hard to grow up.

Another woman was able to let herself be more intimate with a man in the group, and work through with him how neither knew how to love and were terrified of it. Another man, who was compulsive in his life and rigid in his relationships, let himself, after urging from me, become the adorable little boy in the group, something he could never be in his family. Another woman, a longstanding patient, was able to admit how much she loved and adored me, and how I occupied many moments in her fantasy life. Two patients had searing confrontations with their mothers in the group, which freed them to find new men in their lives.

I have had many patients, at great risk to themselves and to our work, get into heated exchanges with me around my technique, or comments I made about their behavior. A patient and I went at it when I confronted her for her thousand times of explaining why she could not get a job. I said, "You prefer being a spoiled brat who wants it both ways, with me and the group. You really enjoy the thrill of it, which I can see on your face, but I'm sick and tired of it. You're not making any progress toward growing up. You're just being a stubborn pain in the ass who still wants my respect and admiration. The only thing I can admire is how you can hold on to your Passionate Bad Fit forever and never tire of it. You can't have it both ways. Get a damn job already and grow up! And you wonder why you are depressed, why you get caught up in difficult issues with your family, have trouble finishing things, and are still unhappy with your life."

She acknowledged that this fight with me was very helpful, because it was a fight she could never have with her father. She felt invigorated by the fight, closer to me, and more aware of the futility of living in the Passionate Bad Fit. I said, "The group and I will keep our hopes for change on the back burner, and we can both hope that you will have the courage to be loved and admired in a healthier way, and use your healthy narcissism to get bigger, and feel really proud of your writing, your daughter, and your ability to curtail your disruptive behavior."

These are all examples of individual group members taking risks, while the group itself also takes risks. Some members cannot borrow my healthy narcissism for themselves, because it feels too intimate and sexual, or too childlike, in wanting the parent to make them bigger. The work of taking risks keeps happening and is integral to my theory and practice.

Part IV

Related Topics

Coming in from the Cold: "Conversation with a Stone"

Pre-Institute Plenary Speech at AGPA February 2016[1]

It's an honor to be asked to give this talk, and a special pleasure because the Institute has played an important part in my personal and professional development. I'm thrilled to be here, and I'm excited to read you a poem by Wislawa Szymborska (1998) called *Conversation with a Stone*.

> *I knock at the stone's front door.*
> *"It's only me, let me come in.*
> *I want to enter your insides,*
> *have a look round,*
> *breathe my fill of you."*
> *"Go away," says the stone.*
> *"I'm shut tight.*
> *Even if you break me to pieces,*
> *we'll all still be closed.*
> *You can grind us to sand,*
> *we still won't let you in."*
> *I knock at the stone's front door.*
> *"It's only me, let me come in.*
> *I've come out of pure curiosity.*
> *Only life can quench it.*
> *I mean to stroll through your palace,*
> *then go calling on a leaf, a drop of water.*
> *I don't have much time.*
> *My mortality should touch you."*
> *"I'm made of stone," says the stone,*
> *"and must therefore keep a straight face.*
> *Go away.*
> *I don't have the muscles to laugh."*
> *I knock at the stone's front door.*
> *"It's only me, let me come in.*
> *I hear you have great empty halls inside you,*
> *unseen, their beauty in vain,*

DOI: 10.4324/9781032705835-17

soundless, not echoing anyone's steps.
Admit you don't know them well yourself."
"Great and empty, true enough," says the stone,
"But there isn't any room.
Beautiful, perhaps, but not to the taste
of your poor senses.
You may get to know me, but you'll never know me through.
My whole surface is turned toward you,
all my insides turned away."
I knock at the stone's front door.
"It's only me, let me come in.
I don't seek refuge for eternity.
I'm not unhappy.
I'm not homeless.
My world is worth returning to.
I'll enter and exit empty-handed.
And my proof I was there
will be only words,
which no one will believe."
"You shall not enter," says the stone.
"You lack the sense of taking part.
No other sense can make up for your missing sense of taking part.
Even sight heightened to become all-seeing
will do you no good without a sense of taking part.
You shall not enter, you have only a sense of what that sense should be,
only its seed, imagination."
I knock at the stone's front door.
"It's only me, let me come in.
I haven't got two thousand centuries,
so let me come under your roof."
"If you don't believe me," says the stone,
"just ask the leaf, it will tell you the same.
Ask a drop of water, it will tell you what the leaf has said.
And, finally, ask a hair from your own head.
I am bursting with laughter, yes, vast laughter,
although I don't know how to laugh."
I knock at the stone's front door.
"It's only me, let me come in."
"I don't have a door," says the stone.

The poem captures the struggle we all experience in our effort to come in from the cold. This inside/outside is portrayed so well in the poem, in which the narrator knocks at the stone's front door and keeps asking, "It's only me. Let me come in," and the recalcitrant stone rebuffs his advances.

I was told many times that I didn't look like anyone in my family, and I imagined that my mother must have had an affair with the milkman, who had the light blonde hair that I had as a kid, and I really felt I didn't belong. But like so many of our patients or clients, I functioned at a high level in spite of myself. I was well liked and relied heavily on a sense of humor and on weaving stories from whatever was being talked about. I was clearly in, as the storyteller, but internally I remained alone and hungry.

I was in analysis when I started my psychiatric training, and then later on, during a difficult marriage. Nothing touched this characterological piece of me, and I was damn glad it didn't. Who else could be so successful living this way and tolerating the loneliness? The self-centered loneliness worked for quite a while, through blaming others and choosing people who would allow me to keep alive my Passionate Bad Fit. I was heroically attached to my magnificence. I made my own lap and by God it was the best in town.

In returning to the poem, we see how powerful the need is for both the narrator and the stone to hold on to their Passionate Bad Fits. The narrator's repetitive and intense yearnings to enter the stone fall on deaf ears. The narrator will not accept the stone's No for an answer. He uses flattery—"You have great empty halls inside of you unseen, their beauty in vain." He uses empathy— "Admit you don't know them well yourself." You see we are both in the same boat. We both need to teach each other about the empty halls. The stone rebuffs the narrator again, and says, basically, nice try but flattery and empathy and attunement won't work. I turn away from you, in spite of your pleadings. The narrator tries another attempt. He says that I won't be much of a bother to your insides, I really am happy and content and I won't make any demands on you that would make you feel uncomfortable. I'll just come and go quickly, like I really wasn't in at all. You don't even have to explain my entrance to anyone, because no one will know, just you and me. It is not enough; the stone doesn't budge; and then the stone really lets the narrator have it—he ridicules his requests by saying he is missing a sense of taking part. The narrator still tries to convince the stone by saying that it is urgent and time is passing by. The narrator, stuck in his own bad fit, refuses to believe the stone. The stone, stuck in his bad fit, tells the narrator to stop pleading with him to have a relationship, to just believe him when he says, "I'm made of stone, and must therefore keep a straight face, go away. I don't have the muscles to laugh." He tells the narrator to check out his own body—"Ask a hair on your own head." It will tell you the truth that I have no door. I think we have all experienced dilemmas like these in our lives and in our groups, and you may notice that you might edge close to repeating this dynamic in your group experiences.

This sad story of the attempt to have a conversation in this poem is a remarkable example of the internal and external dilemmas of the Passionate Bad Fit or the Omnipotent Child. The role and function of the Omnipotent Child is to stabilize identity and serve as a template for intimacy. It dictates how our stories will play out.

We all need to tell our stories. On the new Maya Angelou stamp, there is a quote: "A bird doesn't sing because he has an answer, he sings because he has a song."

We tell our stories because living without telling them is lonely and keeps us out in the cold. Eventually, we hope you decide to sing your song. You do it to attach. You tell your stories, each in your own way. You can tell them with sadness, like a man in my twice-weekly group, who cried during each session for three years before he could believe that, even though he was sad and ashamed, we still loved him. You can tell them with silence, arrogance, seductiveness, bravado, or exuberance. I had a man who for two years called me to complain bitterly about the price of the group before he let himself enter the group. He then stayed for about six years. He eventually was able to understand that his calls to me were his way of telling me that he was a colicky infant. He felt his mother could never understand his distress.

As Jerry Gans (2018) recently wrote, telling his own story, the beauty and wonderment of the unconscious process is that it makes the attachment stronger. I believe that the unconscious moment is really the first true moment of attachment to the process of working through and changing the internal life machinery.

My first moment didn't occur in a group, but instead in my first analysis while I was a resident. After a few months of lying on the analytic couch, I began dreaming of riding in a jeep with the cover blowing over my eyes, in a way that frightened me and made it hard to see. My analyst's response was that there was something in the office that I didn't want to see. The dream recurred often, with no headway in my associations to figure it out, and her responses stayed the same.

One day, while chatting with my fellow residents, one of them asked who my analyst was, and I told him her name. He said, "What's it like to have the only female black training analyst in Boston?" I was shocked, dismayed, and felt a great deal of shame about failing to see what was right in front of me, something I knew a lot about in my personal life. I told my analyst the story of my sudden awareness and could not believe that I couldn't and wouldn't see what was quite apparent. She said, "That has been the story of your life." We laughed together, with a profound sense of mutual relief. We became a team working together at that moment, and I was no longer in the cold alone, in a scary jeep where I couldn't see where I was going, having to live with things out of my control, and feeling helpless. I was hooked as I had never been hooked before. To this day, I find that the dreams and fantasies of group members are crucial in the work.

I was educated to be a physical chemist until I went into the basement of the labs one day and saw the lonely, old, agonized students trying for the hundredth time to get the right result for their PhD experiments. I was in the cold, but not that cold. I went to medical school and found warmth. But in graduate school, I learned about the Heisenberg Uncertainty Principle, which states that you can never simultaneously know the exact position and the exact speed of an object, and I still use it in my mind when dealing with fantasies and dreams, as if they are leaving their trace to tell us about something that happened but couldn't be captured in both time and space. This is the unconscious, the osmotic experience of people putting things into us, whether it is the early mother–infant dyad, or some other projective identification. It is present; we know of it by its trace. We can't ever really see it live; we can only infer its presence. This is the wonder and excitement that I hope we can all provide each other these next two days. Get lost in time and space and notice your fantasies and dreams.

Do we want to witness the insides of our therapist or does he want to view the insides of his patients? I invite people to come inside through the lap, or whatever way they want to enter. I put into words what I think most of us want to say but dare not. What will you want from your Institute group? Do you want to be seen, understood? We all say we do, but most of us don't. Most of us would prefer to live with our exciting Omnipotent Child, our Passionate Bad Fit, and still try to function as well as we can. This Omnipotent Child is our best friend and we are extremely and heroically loyal to that part of us. That part holds all the somatic, passionate misattunements in our bodies and eventually in our thoughts, conflicts, and personalities. A perfect example came from someone in one of my long-term groups when he described how his 5-year-old daughter, who recently had reconstructive facial surgery to remove a congenital abnormality, responded when told how wonderful she looked. She broke into tears and said, "I miss my booboo!" The group burst into laughter and tears saying, "We all want our booboos back. That's why we're all here." We all want to have the best life possible and keep the booboo.

"I'm shut tight," the stone says,
"Even if you break me to pieces
We'll all still be closed.
You can grind us to sand
We still won't let you in."

Why won't the stone let us in? This struggle is what makes the Institutes so great. We all struggle for a piece of each of us. The leaders need you to give them something to make them feel valuable, while the groups feel valuable in having each other. At first, they do not trust each other. Why should they? How are you going to trust each other over this 2-day Institute experience? It makes the work so much easier when we all know that we start in the same place. We all want to be known (up to a point), while each feeling loyal to either our theories or our Passionate Bad Fits. We have to hope that our leaders aren't too loyal to their Passionate Bad Fits.

"You lack the sense of taking part," the stone says.
"No other sense can make up for your missing sense of taking part."

Conversation with a Stone beautifully describes the intense, powerful, intimate attachment that doesn't work. But it is as strong as one that works and, in my way of thinking, is more intense and exciting than the ones that do work. The narrator can only come in when and if he can understand and attune to the "sense of taking part." What does that mean for us as we prepare for our Institutes today and tomorrow? Who do we attend to in the beginning of the group today: the group members, the leaders, or ourselves? As we sit in the group room, do we pay attention to our own anxiety, excitement, fears of failure or exposure, or our own bodies? Are my insides, like the stone's, full of beautiful "great empty halls unseen, their beauty in vain, soundless, not echoing anyone's steps"?

We take part in letting ourselves know the stone in all of us, who won't let anyone in, or the pleading one who tries to do whatever he can to gain admission to the great empty hall. We all want something else, that magnificent moment of merger, that sense of taking part and being one with someone, to fill the empty halls. Even though, like the narrator,

> *"I'm not unhappy.*
> *I'm not homeless.*
> *My world is worth returning to.*
> *And my proof I was there*
> *Will be only words,*
> *Which no one will believe."*

All I want is a moment that someone will understand. It is my basic, earliest body identity that periodically must be attended to, in order to feel alive, to feel me, and to know my own empty spaces. Even when we are maturely attached, the longing for that special moment remains alive and attention has to be paid to it. This is why the therapist's lap must always remain available to all and at all developmental phases in the group.

The human pull to attach and seek a merger will be intense, while at the same time you will want to be left alone.

> *"Just ask the leaf,*
> *Ask a drop of water*
> *And finally ask a hair from your own head."*

Ask the group, the leaders, and yourself why you feel so alone amid a plethora of attachment figures. As the group goes on, you will notice familiar yearnings that are passionate, but not healthy for you, since they keep alive old bad fits. Embrace these bad fits, explore them, and learn who you are and where you came from.

> *I knock at the stone's front door.*
> *"It's only me, let me come in."*
> *"I don't have a door," says the stone.*

What happens when you realize that you don't have a door? What happens when you realize that the person you have been trying to reach does not have a door? Is it a relief, or is it just another moment of agony and despair?

Whichever it is, when you can notice this dilemma, that the quest is impossible, then you will be able to "burst with laughter, yes, laughter, vast laughter, although I don't know how to laugh." This kind of laughter is the laughter of freedom from the heroic grip of the Passionate Bad Fit, and it should be vast and powerful and start you on a path for healthier mature attachments.

When you come into the groups today, you will try, or not try, to tell your story. The story comes out with or without your consent. So don't fight it—surrender and enjoy the space to tell your story. How will I tell my story and to whom? Who will listen, and how can I be assured that I won't feel shame when I tell or refuse to tell? Don't worry; the shame is in all of us, and we just have to worry about whether we get too excited in the shame. I'm sure that all of you, if you take a moment, have found yourselves doing or thinking something shameful and maybe even getting a kick out of it. What is the story that you are going to tell? Will you tell it sooner or later? It's the story about you before you had words. It's like the stone, having or not having a door. It's like the empty halls and how they got filled or never got filled. It's like the shame of not being filled or not filling the other's halls. The bodily feelings of the first attachment and their neurobiological imperatives that get laid down and organize us in our later attachments. The story is about how our identity got laid down in those wordless spaces of body to body and gaze to gaze and mutual laughter at the mystery of it all and the splendor of those delicious moments, like a drop of water on a leaf, or that vast laughter, even though you didn't know what was funny or even knew how to laugh.

How do we do it in the groups? We do it through the members and the leaders. We do it by immediately noticing that we have already picked out someone from whom we want something, or want to rescue. The push to attach is as strong as the push for safety and aloneness. Don't be shy; play with that fantasy, and let yourself feel it, and then notice what comes to your mind and body. Notice whether the leader is seen as interfering with this delicate process or encouraging it to move forward. How does he encourage it?

First of all, we are the best leaders in the country, and, just in case we need help, we have our own source of support from our peer group tables throughout this Institute. So, whether you believe it or not, you don't have to fill us up. We are filled and our halls are not empty. But you will try to rescue us, if this is part of your story. Remember, most of us are rescuers and at the same time need to be rescued. We keep coming back to AGPA to get replenished, to get fed through our relationships of all sizes and styles. No matter what the topic of the institute is, the group dynamics will be there to be examined. You may tell your story through silence, moping, being injured, being grandiose, being shamed, or being hungry. You may not like the group room or the temperature or the noise next door and complain about it as if you are reliving the bad fit in the body space of your mothering figure. These are the early signs of the story of early misattunements, for both the leader and the group. We, the leaders, are not immune to complaining bitterly about our room choices. I, for one, prefer a very special small suite where I can hear the group easily with my hearing aids in place. Thank God I'm not narcissistic or entitled.

Your story may be filled with intense feelings that may surprise others in the group. Your story may be filled with highly intellectual explanations of matters in the group. You may find a corner to hide, you may doze off, you may flirt, or you may be totally obnoxious. All of these characteristic ways of interacting are parts of your early identity that impact your relationships in the group and with the leader. Please let them happen. Bring in your bad fits and your lousy relationships. We don't want you to be on your best behavior, unless that is part of your story as well. The more bad fits you can reenact with us, the more you will be able to laugh at the absurdity of them. And then you can begin to notice the excitement that sits in all of them.

> There is the classic case of a man in one of the groups who continually tried to get a woman in the group to notice him, even though she had categorically stated that she had no interest in him or anyone else in the group. Then there was a single man who, in the group, said that, to his dismay, he had been unable to stop his weekly attempts to sabotage the best relationship he has ever had.

What can we learn from the groups that keep us coming back? Let me recount what my Institute groups taught me. When I decided to work with Dr. Yvonne Agazarian, I wanted to learn what therapist-centered group therapy looked like. Well, I certainly got what I came for. I wanted to be as strong and powerful as she was, and I needed a framework other than systems theory, which didn't appeal to me at all. In my analytic training, the only theoretician that appealed to me was Margaret Mahler. She expressed what I felt about the human condition. I read Mahler (1968) and looked for a way to integrate my own style and personality with her developmental model in my groups. Mahler's theory was based on the importance of the symbiotic mother–child dyad. I believe the therapist is the most important person in the group, and all group members enter as infants. From this, I developed the Omnipotent Child Theory and Practice (2002).

While I was in analytic training, since group therapy was forbidden, I ran groups *sub rosa*. I have always been a rebel, and at times break the rules. I even ate an orange walking past my neighborhood synagogue during a Yom Kippur afternoon break. As you can imagine, my father was furious with me. With his four boys he was highly respected. I took care of that. I was both a good and bad son. I knew I had to deal with power, my own power, and the power of others, healthy power and unhealthy power. I knew about the power of resistance in my patients and the power to stay stuck forever. I knew that no matter who the therapist was, or how long the treatment went on, some people didn't change. I needed to understand the role of power in them, in the groups, and in me. What made them so stuck? What made me so stuck in my isolation and loneliness? I felt and learned that early, pre-verbal damage could not easily be retrieved. I wanted the group to look at me and, through our mutual gaze, recreate the earliest dyad with the symbiotic mother. I thought this was an opportunity to try to replicate what I learned from Dr. Semrad (Mazer & Rako, 1980) in my residency. Through his "tour of the body,"

I saw patients have moments of merger with him, as Mahler had written about. But, I did it with the intensity and conviction of a crazed DeNiro character in *Taxi Driver*—"Look at me. Look at me." At that point, I wasn't exactly sure why the members kept coming back, except to wonder what I was going to do next. But they did. They really wanted help to uncover their Omnipotent Child in their lives and in their groups. The Institutes shaped me, contained me, smoothed me, and helped me be more myself. They taught me enough, so I could more easily help the groups to re-enact their earliest, pre-verbal symbiotic phase. Over time, some have commented that I have grown breasts instead of being so phallic. These groups, along with my patients and my wife, have transformed me into being a therapist and a person I really like, respect, and can take seriously. The key for all of us is to take ourselves seriously as therapists, since we have enormous responsibilities to perform on a daily basis. We must have integrity, must keep learning, and keep returning to the best place I know for learning how to be a group therapist. In medical school, and in the emergency room, I was taught about medical procedures that had to be done: See one, do one, and then teach one. At the AGPA, the saying is: join a group, lead a group, and then teach group.

I truly hope that your work in the Institutes this weekend will deepen your healthy excitement in knowing yourselves, and enjoyment in being able to live in the more mature, healthy Passionate Good Fits. They may not be as exciting and thrilling as the bad fits, but the warmth, companionship, and trust light up the sky. Every year for me it is a renewal of old pleasures, old friendships, and a sense of taking part as someone with both feet in. The Institute, over time, became a home to me. It gave me a place where my loneliness and isolation could turn into healthy connections and empathy for myself and others. It helped me find a lap to rest in and then to build one for others, something my individual analysis rarely did. I envy all of you today.

Note

1 Reprinted from the *International Journal of Group Psychotherapy*, 67, 597–606, ©2017 The American Group Psychotherapy Association, Inc reprinted by permission of Taylor & Francis Ltd, http://www.tandfonline.com on behalf of The American Group Psychotherapy Association, Inc.

Chapter 14

Character Change
and Narcissism

The parameters of character change have shifted over the years, as the models of intrapsychic and interpersonal theory have changed. In the early classical psychoanalytic models, the resolution of the transference neuroses was the *sine qua non* of character change. This was basically a resolution of oedipal issues and tended to ignore the pre-oedipal issues. As ego psychology came into prominence, the shift toward ego functions and pre-oedipal issues became more manifest as the conflict-free areas of the ego propelled investigators to expect more from themselves and their patients. Everyone was to go deeper and pay more attention to object relations.

The shift to object relations propelled the debate to include not only the resolution of the drive-seeking intrapsychic conflicts but also the interpersonal object-seeking drives and, equally important, the projective identifications that reside in the ego and superego. Character change then became the working through of these identifications as they related to the distortions of reality testing in the patient's view of themselves and his expectations of the course and shape of his relationships. If one could uncover these early identifications, and then take them back and grieve them, then character change would occur and the capacity for mature relationships would blossom.

Kohut (1978) and the self psychologists then went a bit further, when they worked with the narcissistic lines of normal and abnormal development and postulated a deficit model of intrapsychic development. In this model, character change occurs when the patient is able to work through, in the transference, the narcissistic distortions, and put into the system what had been missing from early on in the dyad. In this process, the patient learns to tolerate frustrations better and reclaims what was his and tolerates stronger affects, as there is more self inside now.

The interpersonal model relies on the object-seeking drives and pushing the patient to work through conflicts in the here-and-now in the group, where deepening personal disclosures about each other (including the therapist) lead to character change and more intimate relationships.

In my updated model of intensive therapist-centered group psychoanalysis, character change is produced through working through of the many developmental cycles with their attendant narcissistic injuries, defenses, and entitlements. Each

DOI: 10.4324/9781032705835-18

phase of life recapitulates the earliest developmental changes that Mahler (1968) and Pine (1985) described so beautifully. There is the wish for and fear of merger, the need to hatch with its attendant anxieties of loss of the loved one, castration, loss of self, and containing excitement. There is the absolutely necessary state of rapprochement, where one can attempt to find a safe shelter and fix what is broken, and then proceed to go out again, only to repeat the cycles with different people and different ego skills and different psychic internal structures. My postulation is that, within each phase of development, there is the potential for a good or a bad fit that defines the narcissistic proclivities of the psyche and the parameters of the relationships. The good fit allows the dyad to grow, heal, and be soothed and neutralizes inherent aggression in the psyche. It leads to a sense of well-being, and hence a potential for creativity and a sense of being able to tolerate strong affects. It leads to a sense of optimism and certainty in life. The bad fit leads to insecurity, un-neutralized aggression, negativity about the future of relationships, and a flourishing of the Omnipotent Child with all its attendant problems. Its hallmark is the search for the great moment and the inevitable catastrophic landing. It leads to recreating bad fits and projecting into others the bad introjects. One expects injury and lack of healing as a way of life. Rapprochement offers a chance for healing and correction of the bad fits, hence the function of our therapy groups. We work in the phase of rapprochement a great deal to effect character change.

In this model, a clear distinction is made between *symptom improvement* and *character change*. Symptom improvement allows the work to go deeper as it strengthens and increases the conflict-free sphere of the ego for more work. Lurking in the deep recesses, the narcissistic moments of bad fits remain basically untouched until the earlier work is done in the therapeutic alliance, resolution of important conflicts, symptom improvement, and the patient's sense that there is something better out there than his own system. Many therapists and patients stop at this point because the patient is feeling better, his life looks healthier, and the therapist is feeling very successful. Agazarian, 1997 said that when the patient says he is ready to go that we should agree. Not in my approach, because in the body of work that has transpired, you can see and experience many of the bad fits that are still in place but didn't get worked through in the transferences to the therapist, to the group as a whole, and to the individual members. This is where character change takes place.

There are at least four major points of narcissistic bad fits that must be worked through to enable a new character structure to emerge: (1) the very obvious entitlements and narcissistic defenses; (2) the Omnipotent Child, with its full, powerful affects and fantasies that must be explored fully; (3) the struggle to contain and fully experience excitement and arousal in the transference and the struggle with being envied; and (4) the struggle with the preverbal influences on the repetition compulsion.

The culture has to allow regressive behavior and strong affects to exist to allow the bad fits to develop as a way to understand them, as well as a way to transform them. There is a very narcissistic patient in one of my groups who refuses to bend to the group's will and become a patient, not a therapist, and experiences the group as a bad fit, yet keeps on coming to wait out the group until they surrender to her. When she allows herself for a moment to drop her protest and merge with the group, she is actually comforted. So, in my group, scapegoating and isolation have to exist and are not considered harmful to the treatment but essential for the character's work to go on.

I will in the beginning of treatment try to define what kind of fit the patient needs to enable the work to occur. I will suggest to patients that they need me to be a bad mother, or a seductive father, or a sadistic parent in order to feel that there is a place for their history and their internalized projections to appear. This is also an important aspect of trust, and nurturing, since the patient can now be at home. The therapist doesn't act out, and when he does it usually explodes in his face.

> A new patient in my twice-weekly group called me to tell me she was pregnant and couldn't tell the group, because she had to make up her own mind if she was going to keep the child. I went along with this, and therefore collaborated with her need to have a sexy secret, which later we were to learn was a replication of her dirty secret of sexual abuse. My collaborating with her secret was fueled by her tenuous grasp in the group, as well as my failure to notice the narcissistic elements and grandiosity in the wish to do it alone. I let myself be blackmailed to avoid her narcissistic rage. She didn't last in the group, but now has returned.

If the therapy is seen as a continual recycling of the developmental stages, then we have multiple chances to work thorough the bad fits and explore them at each cycle and at each separate phase of the cycle. Throughout this exploration, there is a great deal of aggressive affect that is released, as well as momentary feelings of relief that there is a possibility of something different.

> In one group, we have three people who are constantly and chronically stuck in their lives, and they would rather rail at the narcissistic woman than look at those narcissistic entitlements in themselves. The bulk of the work is to let them know how they hold onto their "catbird seat" of despair. When they are confronted, a storm of anger or hurt feelings erupts. I am not dismayed, and cannot be. I let them know how entitled they are, and how stingy they are to others in their life and in the group, and how ultimately boring they are in their insistence on their unique, exquisite catbird seat.

It takes time, and must be repeated, and then explored, and then empathized with, and then listened to again, and retraced through their genetic histories and their transference histories in the group. You contain your own narcissistic injuries and failures of your own Omnipotent Child. You explore the origins of the bad fits, you explore the Omnipotent Child that sits behind this position, and the sad bankruptcy of their positions, and how painful it is to take the next step.

The fear of the unknown is certainly present, but in my experience it is related to accepting that what you have built your life on is a failure, like suddenly realizing that you put all your money in the wrong bank, and you kept on doing it. How stupid, how foolish, how awful. To breach the unknown, you have to tolerate the most painful, narcissistic injury, to imagine yourself with a new set of basic assumptions, and to tolerate powerful feelings of being full, full of pleasure, excitement, and power—to go from bad fits to good fits. While this storm is going on, very subtle changes are occurring in the transferences and in the patient's behavior inside and outside the group room. Different decisions are made, and the relief of the aggression being neutralized by the copious tears of empathy and sadness for the mistakes of life and the bad luck of life and bad genes of life is enormously gratifying. Someone, for the first time, decides to get a job that he really wants; someone decides for the first time that she wants to leave her self-imposed cloister and start her life; someone gets a facelift and starts dating women; and a woman one day will yield to the group and merge with us, rather than insisting that we merge with her.

Chapter 15

Impasse

Impasse is not failure. Impasse occurs when the group is stuck around an issue between members that feels as if it cannot be resolved and can dangerously lead to dissolution of the group or the fleeing of a member.

Impasse is also present within the therapist, when he is struck with intolerable feelings toward the group or members of the group. This leads to silence, work not being done, or acting out on the part of the therapist, which in itself can lead to destruction of the group or the scapegoating of one member to rescue the stuck and ineffective therapist.

Impasse can also be felt and experienced when the working theoretical model cannot take care of the issues at hand in the group and in the therapist. The group may slow down, work may stop, the group may start to feel boring or passive, and patient and therapist lose interest in the work and certainly in the passion of the group.

I know when impasse occurs because I feel angry and don't want the problematic patients to stay in the group. I recognize it also when I lose interest in going to group, and I feel dread and want to stay away. I also know I'm in an impasse when I regress to earlier moments of my life that I passionately hated, and still can feel that taste in my mouth.

In my theoretical framework, impasse occurs when the group and a patient's Omnipotent Child collide and there is the feeling that there is no give. It is experienced as lose–lose. What is at stake is a newer, healthier identity and a different template for intimacy, both of which are experienced as major terrifying losses. The following case really puts the spotlight on this Omnipotent Child impasse.

The drama of Charley and Al, over time, has touched on all the above aspects of impasse, which led me and the group to powerfully passionate moments that have changed the culture of the group, and saved one member and lost another. Therapist disclosure of the issues, in the group and in the therapist, were crucial to this resolution. The notion of the Passionate Bad Fits or Omnipotent Child exposed itself in various disguises that got illuminated over time.

DOI: 10.4324/9781032705835-19

Charley had been in the group for about 16 years. He was a volatile person who couldn't work regularly for the last 10 years, even though he had previously. He usually quit or was fired or flunked out of jobs and career situations prior to the group. He was narcissistic, depressed, and infantile in his behavior and in his quixotic moods and entitlement issues. During the group work, he tried different work experiences, only to leave quickly when faced with tough decisions. He did get married, and I encouraged that, even though we all knew it was a difficult Passionate Bad Fit. I believed he needed to move on, even though it wasn't the best choice. The marriage did not work and we dealt with his loss. It foundered over whether they could have a baby. He backed out.

Charley was well liked in the group, in spite of his outbursts. He felt to me like the group's mascot. The group hid their Passionate Bad Fits in loving the child Charley. I began over the years to really dislike his childlike behavior, like bringing in a cute little hat to wear to group that made him look idiotic. I told him to get rid of it. We felt close to each other, he idealized me at times, yet kept his relationship very much superficial, rather than deal with the fantasies. He was terrified over homosexual longings, which sometimes occurred in the group.

All of that was tolerable, and I kept thinking that one day he could make a change and be more adult. Then Al entered the group, and all hell broke out from the very beginning. Al couldn't stand Charley's arrogance dominating the room, nor his special role of therapist in the group. Their competition to be my favorite child undermined them both. Neither could deal with that interpretation and exploration. Fights would break out; they would each provoke the other, and the group room became a vicious, heavyweight battle between them, with everyone making efforts to calm them down and, at the same time, unconsciously rooting for Charley to vanquish Al. What was remarkable was the group's total adoration and support of Charley and his childlike behavior, while being totally unsupportive of Al's contemptuous and devaluing behavior. There was an impasse within the group, between the group and Al and Charley, between Charley and Al, and between the group and the leader.

I wanted them both to leave the group. Al openly struggled with leaving the group, but didn't want to give up because he wanted to keep alive his hope that therapy could be helpful, not hurtful, even though he felt that the group was punishing and hurtful. The group, in fact, had chosen him as the villain, not Charley. But he couldn't see his role in the scapegoating. To say that they were both reenacting their chaotic childhoods with each other is an understatement. No interpretation or insight would stop them. I explained to the group Al's struggle with holding the group in contempt on numerous occasions when he wouldn't come to group. He did take some solace in seeing me individually, which Charley had done previously in his own work with the group. The similarities in their struggle and their relationship to the group were remarkable, but each expressed it in his own way. Neither felt they could capture the elusive or difficult father (therapist).

To resolve the issue, I strongly suggested that Charlie get a job within three months. This would be consistent with my model of the therapist's activity in the group. The decision was explained in depth, and my feelings of frustration with Charley were further emphasized over time. That led to Charley leaving the group two sessions later without saying goodbye to the group.

The internal work of the therapist and the group that followed was remarkable. I found myself more open with my internal workings than ever before, and the group's maturation increased as well, seeing how other members now took over the resistant and frustrating positions in the group. Much healthier intimacy occurred among all of us, and the Omnipotent Child was equally shared including mine. What happened, and was it for the good of the group? Or for the therapist, or even for Charley or Al? Only time will tell.

Al has quieted down without Charley in the room, and is only now beginning to look at his role in the scapegoating, even though he still struggles over whether he will leave the group, and when. This is a good example of a group enabling Charley to not grow and to protect themselves from their own failures and inadequacies, while the same group didn't give Al a break as he became the hated pre-oedipal mother in their life who was beating up on them, especially Charley. It was also a painful and needed reminder of the power of the Passionate Bad Fit and how monumental it is. The group needed to look at what living in this bad fit is costing them. They needed to see where their lives have stopped developmentally, and where it had stopped in the group, and how it was much more exciting to be in the bad fit than to move on in their lives. We all moved on, but the child and the pre-oedipal mother needed the father to step in and end the impasse.

Chapter 16

It Takes Courage to Live in a Good Fit

Recent psychoanalytic literature and the resurgence of attachment theory have brought back into focus the influence of good and bad fits. Simply put, good fits occur when the earliest experiences of infancy, between mother and infant, are mutually satisfying. Does the mother know what the baby needs? Does she know how to soothe the baby? Does she allow the baby to turn away from her, allow the baby to meet its own need to not be overstimulated? Can she regulate both her own internal life and the child's internal and external life, so that the child feels safe and attached to a mothering figure who appreciates his uniqueness from others? The healthier the mothering figure, the easier and more natural these tasks of early childhood become.

These early good and bad fits can, at times, have a disproportionate influence on the child's relationship to others, the role of intimacy, his relationship to his body, and, most importantly, his sense of identity. When there are good fits, the child is able to be optimistic in his life, attach to a healthier person, be more curious, take healthy risks, and feel as if his body is an ally, not an enemy that needs to be punished. Bad fits of early childhood leave the child with feelings of inadequacy, despair, fear of life, a profound distrust of his body, lack of curiosity with the world, and a tendency to assume the worst in relationships. His identity is marked by a yearning for closeness, without an ability to master the art of attachment.

These good and bad fits are filled with strong somatic affects and excitement that tend to lay down neuronal pathways in the brain. These passions imbue the child with an excitement that continually leads to the repetition of both these good and bad fits. These re-enactments stabilize the early sense of self in identity and in the body. Such moments all lead to lifetime templates of intimacy.

Jane experiences a healthier relationship for the first time. She begins to feel dread and anxiety as she recognizes her strong desire to reject her new lover. Her anxiety touches the loss of her old identity. She dreads losing a familiar, bad-fit intimacy. She becomes aware, through dreams and dream associations, that being with her new lover is a new excitement but, at the same time, she feels she could disappear into a black hole, feeling lost and unprotected without any identity.

DOI: 10.4324/9781032705835-20

The intense combination of new, highly charged excitement in a relationship is often coupled with anxiety and dread over the loss of an old identity. Such anxiety is the hallmark of the transition from a bad to good fit. Our task is to help the patient understand how it takes courage to live in the good fit. The bad fits call and echo an enticing familiarity. The patient, through his analytic work, must find the courage to explore his dilemma—to stay in the old bad fit, or to move on to the new good fit. It takes courage to withstand the powerful call of the bad fit. As the new identity emerges, it may even get harder for the patient.

Patients will go to all lengths to maintain their Omnipotent Child in order to stabilize their earlier identity. They will start eating after weight-loss surgery; they will lose a job; they will become much more anxious and outrageous; and they will test the group and demand they be thrown out. Some will eroticize the transition and demand that the group be seduced by them. They will act out. They will return to older, bad-fit relationships with the group and other people in their lives. The group can also become Nitsun's (1996, 2006) anti-group. The therapist must continue to interpret to the group their struggle to live in the good fit and explore with them all the issues involved in this transition. In this context, the acting out has a better chance to be managed. The most important comments the therapist can make are to acknowledge that the passion of the good fit may never match the intensity of the passion of the bad fit. Through this hard work, one discovers the power of self-righteous indignation and its influence in relationships and in the development of holding on to the Passionate Bad Fit. The powerful need to build a monument to the Passionate Bad Fit unfolds with all its grandiosity and magnificence within the group work to transition to a Passionate Good Fit. The therapist must encourage the monument building for this transition to move along. The patient then has to look at his ability to build the monument, so he can live in the heroic Passionate Bad Fit until he realizes what price he pays.

Chapter 17

Excitement

A Crucial Marker for Group Psychotherapy[1]

Introduction

In 2002, I developed the construct of the Omnipotent Child to describe the role of the Passionate Bad Fits in the formation of identity and the laying down of templates of intimacy (Aledort, 2009). As such, the Omnipotent Child contains high-intensity, somatic affect. Bad fits can occur from misattunements in early childhood, or any subsequent developmental phase. Here I look at the role of excitement in the formation, stabilization, and resolution of the Omnipotent Child, or Passionate Bad Fits, as its focus of attention. Excitement is a high-intensity, somatic affect not synonymous with pleasure, though it can be pleasurable and highly eroticized. All conflict situations, whether intrapsychic or interpersonal, are sources of excitement. Excitement is an integral part of all developmental phases from infancy to adulthood.

Infant studies from Beebe (2000) and Stern (1985) confirm that serious problems occur in attachments, and hence development, when there is either too much or too little stimulation. They underscore the role of intense affect in creating the strongly held misattunements in pre-verbal relationships. The potency of these strong affects is such that at times it cannot escape repetition. Repetitious reenactment of these bad fits can be an attempt at mastery over injured ego states (Hendrick, 1943), or an effort to stabilize the sense of self-identity (Cohen, 2000; Schermer, 2000; Stolorow & Lachman, 1980). The Omnipotent Child is another construct that attempts to stabilize the core self, even if it is in a Passionate Bad Fit. I believe that the remarkable stability and repetitious nature of these bad fits are the result of the hidden excitement in them.

When we turn our attention to the literature on group therapy, there has been scant discussion on the influence of excitement. Rosenthal (2006) talks of excitement in the process of role reenactments in the group, saying that these roles were fixed from early family experiences and that these roles stir up intense affect in the group. Ormont (2006) goes further, saying strong emotions are needed to keep the group flourishing and progressing. Livingston's (2003, 2004) focus is on the intense emotion in the vulnerable moments, while Segalla (1996) emphasizes the affect in the formation and stabilization of the self in the group. Livingston (2006)

DOI: 10.4324/9781032705835-21

discusses the importance of recognizing the therapist's affects in acknowledging the presence of shame. Mahler's (1968) developmental model spells out the intra-psychic conflicts and affects in the natural evolution of separation–individuation from the mothering figure. She emphasizes the merged, symbiotic, early pre-verbal phase. Using this model, I detail the role of excitement in each stage.

Phillips (1993) describes feelings of vulnerability in the tickling situation. With tickling, there is a need for a healthy regulation of the vulnerability. Without this, pleasure can easily become pain, or the shame of helplessness at the hands of an-other. Are they the twin feelings that make up the merged experience and contrib-ute to its powerful seductive quality, as well as to its character-changing moment? These feelings of vulnerability (pleasure with the risk of losing oneself, being made more vital and bigger, being inside each other) are crucial, exciting moments. They carry the magic of the merged experience. These moments are the equivalent of the "moments of merger" of Pine (1985), and the "now moments" that Stern (1985) and the Boston Change Group (1998) describe. Psycho-neurological evidence (Kandel, 1998; Kernberg, 2001; Schore, 2002b) supports the hypothesis that those moments may lead to the formation of new neuronal pathways. Continuing stud-ies in this area may eventually demonstrate that some intense experiences become hard-wired in the brain but perhaps can be altered if corrective experiences provide sufficiently powerful and exciting experiential alternatives.

Excitement and the Omnipotent Child in Group Psychotherapy

It is not enough to have reenactments of injury, repair, and empathetic attunement to move toward character change, a new template of intimacy, and a new identity. One must discover, and examine in great detail, the hidden excitement in the old bad fit, in its re-enactment within the group, and in the anxiety-ridden process of repair and replacement. In exploring this process, I take the liberty of using some playful and imaginative constructs, because these are terms that seem to engage group members and help them illuminate hidden and subtle processes that shape their unsatisfying relationships.

The first concept relates to the subjective sense of power attached to the Om-nipotent Child introject. In the group, this is presented as a sense of "fullness" and "bigness," as contrasted with a sense of emptiness, helplessness, and smallness. Patients often try to convince themselves (and the group leader) that there is no feeling of bigness involved in clinging to the bad fit and its repetition. "After all, they argue, I'm here to stop my neurotic behavior." These are truthful statements, since the patient is usually unaware of the excitement attached to feeling big. It is this hidden excitement that perpetuates the pattern. As this unfolds, the therapist begins to comment on the hidden satisfaction in the feelings that accompany the appearance of the Omnipotent Child in the group.

The most glorious of these feelings is self-righteous indignation, though gran-diosity, competitiveness, and seductiveness also appear. Patients may restrain and justify these feelings, as well as their resulting behaviors, since the emergence of the Omnipotent Child carries not only power, but danger. Patients may feel that their fullness cannot be contained. They worry it will be a source of humiliation and shame because the feelings are too intense. They are concerned that their envy, grandiosity, competitiveness, or sexuality will be too powerful for the therapist and the group to tolerate and contain. Others feel they will be too needy, as their feelings of fullness reside in their neediness. Their identity resides in being needy. To them, giving up the old bad-fit identities is the equivalent of being annihilated. Others are concerned they cannot trust themselves enough to explore their dreams and fantasies in the group. It is the therapist's task to provide a safe environment and sufficient stimulation to allow the excitement attached to the bad fit to be expressed and explored within the group.

Group members struggle to grasp the metaphorical concept of using the group leader's lap to provide safety and the opportunity to experience regressive states. Some group members even use the imagery of going into the therapist's insides. The group leader can encourage intense fantasy interactions within the group and the free play of imagery and imagination. All of these techniques are discussed in more detail later.

I will now focus on clinical material to illustrate how different phases in the group therapy process, and in the personal developmental history of each member, are related to the process of unearthing and exploring the excitement accompanying each patient's Omnipotent Child. All therapy groups described are open-ended in their structure. I expand on Mahler's phases of development but subscribe to the current notion that these phases are best used as indicators to help the therapist more fully understand what is going on in the group (Rutan, Stone, & Shay, 2007).

The Impact of the New Patient

The prospect of a new member fills the group leader and group members with strong feelings. Everyone anticipates the advent of the new patient with a multitude of fears, wishes, and hopes that mobilize a great deal of excitement. Group members have many questions. What if they know the new member? Does the intruder have the right to be in the group? Is the new person worthy of membership? Will the new member be a special friend or a hated opponent?

The anticipation of a new member often opens a powerful and rich vein of exciting experiences in many group members. This is one source of group stimulation that sets the stage for the more open appearance of the Omnipotent Child within. The group's anxiety emerges around the wish and fear that the new person will stir up intense erotic or angry feelings in the group. I label the intense anxieties as *excitement*. This begins to lay the groundwork for understanding the concept of the hidden excitement in their anxiety. I encourage the group to attend to these feelings that are inside the therapist and the group. I help the group members use these excited feelings to explore all avenues of excitement that are connected to waiting for changes in the group. Waiting for a phone call, a letter, magic, birth of a sibling, or other events that promise to evoke major change—they all may emerge as a new member's arrival into the group is anticipated. One can learn a great deal from how the individuals and the group negotiate this period of expectation. One can hear family myths and feelings about the birth of group members. Were they, or their siblings, wanted? Stories of disappointment and frustration occur when pleasant anticipation turns ugly.

The Entrance of a New Member

Bert had a difficult entry into his group. He waited six months for an opening. Then, due to a failure in communication, his arrival was not properly announced to the group. The therapist repeatedly apologized for the error. The group was accommodating and welcoming. However, none of this helped Bert. He was furious. He said he felt like a skunk at a party. His fury continued well into the next several sessions. He mentioned that the situation was particularly painful, since his birth had been welcomed by his mother, but not by his father. The group recognized that Bert was revealing something important about his early life.

The intensity of his excitement around entering the group, and his strongly held need to see me as uncaring, despite my subsequent behavior, perplexed the other group members. Bert was helped to recognize how intensely he was organized around his early, unfortunate injury of not being welcomed by his father, and its accidental repetition in the group. Bert was gradually able to examine his excitement in not being cared for. As he stepped back, he was able to see exactly how he got into these exciting struggles with his wife. He realized that these re-enactments with the group, and with his wife, were his passionate struggles to be injured and rejected. They were not struggles to be noticed and loved by his father. The real hidden excitement that had to be analyzed for Bert to change was not the repetitive, bereft longing for rapprochements, but Bert's self-righteous indignation. Bert's Omnipotent Child was to see how many ways he could be injured and therefore justify his continuing to live in self-righteous indignation.

The ongoing group work gave Bert ample opportunity to recognize the internal excitement and fullness he gained by seizing on every perceived slight or rejection. As he gradually gave up his exciting indignation, he was able to begin to live in a good fit with the caring group and the supportive therapist. He became an active member, eagerly, though anxiously, exploring new ways to relate.

Larry's Entry

Larry called me four times to make an appointment. Each time he argued over the rules of the group, the fees, and the meeting times. While the bickering annoyed me, Larry was showing his intimate Omnipotent Child. After four months of calls, Larry finally joined the group. By now I knew that the group's new "baby" would probably be colicky and hard to satisfy. The work in the beginning of the group was to be sensitive to Larry's early Passionate Bad Fit. With some prompting from me, the group heard the origin of this dynamic as he told about his early experiences. The rapidity with which Larry launched into his early bad fits suggested that he was waiting for a safe harbor to tell his story. Larry's early story was the beginning of a long group experience during which he explored his passionate attachment to his Omnipotent Child. His Omnipotent Child identity defined him as being in a state of masochistic surrender. The group recognized the hidden passion in his bad fit. This was primarily expressed through his upper body movements, hidden smiles, grinning, and seductive tears. He reluctantly, but proudly, admitted how he stalemated his previous therapist for years. They were either going to kill each other or end the therapy. The hidden, secret passion of these early bad fits had to be explored. If not, the repetitive injuries and possibility for repair became more hopeless and frustrating to both parties.

How did the group know it was being excited in this experience with Larry? Larry was able to command the attention of the group. His stories were filled with strong affect. The group's responses to him were affectively laden with surprise, curiosity, or laughter. He was infectious in his pathology and the group, in turn, infected him. The group itself was being seductive. At the same time, it was seduced by the energy of Larry's stories and bad fits. Larry never imagined he could be so aroused. His previous experiences always felt so deadening. The merged experience with the group illuminated and underscored the hidden pleasure in Larry's need for masochistic surrender. Larry felt relief when I suggested that perhaps he could be excited with the group without all the agony. The moments of high affect that were shared in the group became the focus for healthy moments of merger (Pine, 1985). The experience of merger, with its excitement in the pleasure of being emotionally held, reduced the impact of the bad fit and encouraged the beginnings of the new, better, healthier fit. These moments of affective merger helped to redo the earlier bad fits of infancy. They pushed the group to further explorations of better fits, with all their attendant resistances, defenses, and joyous discoveries.

The Fit, the Lap, and the Symbiotic Mother

The revelations and the working through of the excitement of the preverbal period were crucial for the establishment of a good-enough analytic culture in order to produce character change and identity shifts. I described this period in great detail in my previous articles (Aledort, 2002, 2003). The crux of this period in the work was how I interpreted and worked with the usual patterns of fight/flight typically seen in group work. In this model, the unfolding of these urges was viewed as stories being told by each group member about their preverbal experiences. The room became the metaphor for the early body of the mother–child dyad. Complaints were registered and remembered. The storytelling, even the flight away, or sleeping, coming late, or leaving the door open, were not seen as resistance to the work, but rather as more information about their pre-verbal experiences. Group members complained of over-stimulation, under-stimulation, not being fed properly, being fed too much, things not fitting right, things being too tight, too cold, too hot, too bright, or too dark in the room. They got angry when I insisted on interpreting their complaints as telling how uncomfortable they felt in their early fits with their mothering figure, and how these complaints organized aspects of their idea of themselves. They tended to get furious when the passion in their complaints was interpreted as the passion of the bad fit. How can a therapist be so unsympathetic to their complaints? How can I be so cold to their pleas for something better?

In this phase, the therapist must contend with his own narcissistic positions, grandiosity, and other feelings. He must contain, inside of himself, the excitement of being the most important person in the room. He must contain his feelings of shame and injury around this role.

To promote the growth of the mother–infant or group–individual dyad, the bigness of the therapist must be present and acknowledged. The importance of regulating the therapist's bigness, excitement, self-centeredness, and responsibility is similar to the passion of a mother regulating her self-centeredness, anxieties, excitements, pleasures, and need to meet the corresponding regulation of the infant's needs. Fonagy (1999) says that co-regulation was defined as behavior that was unfolding in an individual while simultaneously being modified by the changing behavior of a partner. These processes were mostly non-verbal, but the powerful excitements in these mutual interactions led to, and sustained, the co-regulation. These were the moments of merger that carried a continual, mutual unconscious flow of somatic affective information that transformed and initiated emotional and perhaps even neuronal growth.

How does the therapist know when the Passionate Good Fit merged experience takes place? Moments of merger in the group were noted when two people riveted their eyes on each other. Both parties felt special to each other. It was like a cocoon being built around two people. Amazingly, the rest of the group protected the new cocoon through their engaged silence. Once the cocoon was broken, the group worked with their reactions to the moment of merger. The merged pair felt a physical alertness, sometimes eroticized, but more animated and vital. They ultimately felt satisfied, embraced by a shared smile, or shared sadness. Generally in a merger, there are fears of losing oneself. In this merger, the risk was in feeling fuller and bigger. Hence, there was a beginning of excitement and fullness in being able to appreciate being in a good fit.

Eva and a Good Merger

At the end of a session, Eva and I had a moment of merger. She was grateful to me for my help in greatly improving her life. I reminded Eva that we did this together. She looked astonished, then sad. She was like a little girl who was excited but didn't know what to do with her excitement in the good merger. I felt close to her, wanted to hug her, and felt like the two of us had shared something special.

Eva impulsively skipped her next session and visited a hostile and demeaning aunt in another city. She called me three times to say how bad she felt with this wicked aunt. Upon her return, the group focused on how hard it was for her to hold the exciting good fit, and how she needed to return to her familiar, exciting, hurtful bad fit. How many times did I feel, after a long difficult day, the beautiful feeling of being made alive and vibrant through the evening group hour? These moments represented the uplifting feeling of a good fit, which supplies energy, creativity, and life to the group and the therapist. After a particularly difficult session, I applauded my group. I told them that together they did a masterful job and everyone should feel proud. The session ended on that note.

Once the bad fit was identified, and the hidden excitement in the conflict was explored, the group and I engaged in healthier fits. This put a different lens on impasse, resistance, and defenses in the group. The task, then, of this first phase includes: the co-regulation of the group and therapist; the storytelling of the early good and bad fits; and the awareness of the somatic and non-verbal components of the interaction. These were possible because of the ever-present symbiotic mother–therapist who held and contained the group of "infants."

When I was a first-year resident I had to present a patient to the esteemed Dr. Elvin Semrad. The patient was a manic 16-year-old girl who had difficulty controlling her impulses. After the presentation, she jumped eagerly and excitedly into Dr. Semrad's lap and proudly proclaimed that she had finally found the real Santa Claus and hugged him deeply. He looked at her, smiled, and glowed, as he said that he enjoyed the hug. It was exciting to be so close and at one with each other. This was my first lesson about the vicissitudes of excitement—being in the lap, being able to tolerate the closeness of merger, handling the excitement of having someone emotionally enter you, and being whatever they wanted you to be at this moment of merger. Of course, in group work, the therapist's lap is a metaphor. Not everyone can safely be Dr. Semrad.

June and a Good Merger

June, a new member of the group, was overwhelmed and frightened by the intensity of the group. Over the last three months, the group was in the throes of losing two important members. The last member to leave was seen as the "good mother," who calmed the group and enjoyed the mutual excitement of loving and being loved by the therapist. The group felt bereft at being left with the prickly "witch mother," who claimed to be the only fertile female in the group. This member refused to merge with the group and held on to her Omnipotent Child tenaciously. This mirrored for June her own traumatic history of being stuck, as an adolescent, with her depressed mother after both her father and brother died. June's response to this state of affairs was fear, anxiety, and dread. It felt too stimulating, too angry, too reckless, and too close to home for her. She talked of fleeing the group, but resisted, knowing that she could benefit from this experience. I locked eyes with June, feeling her strong emotions. These mirrored my strong feelings about the group's intensity. There was hatred, rage, and sadness in the group. June and I looked at each other for long periods of time in the sessions. Eventually I told her that the two of us needed to keep looking at each other while the rest of the group worked out their feelings. These moments with June were like microsecond soothing interactions of the infant and mother (Stern, 1985). The merger with June lasted 3–5 sessions and gave her and me an opportunity to relax and regulate the ongoing chaos into more livable, yet strong affects. I then turned to other group members and helped them work through their issues while June was able to stay, and continued to feel safe in the eyes of the regulating "good mother." The group accepted the merger between June and me. It helped them talk about their own merged experiences in the group, as well as their longing for the earlier merged moments.

The Body and Separation–Individuation (Hatching)

The next stage of excitement is the period of *discovering the body* and the other. If this period of development goes well, the group member can develop optimism about life, human relationships, and his body. Conversely, if this period has too much impingement, avoidance, or over-stimulation in the dyad (Beebe & Lachman, 2002), maladaptive behaviors of aggression and excessive erotic energy are seen. Trust begins with trusting your own body, and the Omnipotent Child can easily interfere with this process.

In the group, there was an increase in the excitement of the exploration of the dream world. The discovery of the unconscious paralleled the discovery of the body and the beginnings of ownership of the self. In this phase, the group and I focused more on the excitement of discovery than the content of the dreams. Exciting moments of unconscious discoveries took place.

> Rob was a wonderful example of discovery. One day he entered group with a great smile, and a pipe like my pipe. He was excited and ashamed about copying me, not only with the pipe, but with hand movements and facial gestures. I told Rob how delighted I was that he could be close to me, and now played with him, through dream work, without Rob's usual provocative, aggressive grin. Rob's Omnipotent Child in his early work with the group was personified by his frightening the group with tales of being mistreated by a sadistic lover. When he understood how exciting it was for him to frighten us, the way his father frightened him, he changed and modified his behavior. Later, as he sought a healthy mate, and tried to internalize a good fit with me, he continued to feel uneasy. It was not easy to move into a good fit. He noticed his passion was less intense in the healthier relationship. He missed the excitement attached to frightening others and having them frighten him. Rob explored his difficulty in living in a good fit. Over time Rob assumed the role of co-therapist. The group was envious and angry at his position of being in a good fit. Rob was able to tolerate the group's feelings because the merger with me gave him enough strength and courage to withstand the pull to return to the old, passionate bad fit.

During work in this phase, stories of shame and humiliation appeared. Many were related to bosses, spouses, parents, but some involved group members' fantasies.

The members discussed their experiences of discovery, anticipation, magic, and curiosity, which were met with disapproval and shame. I, at this time, gingerly approached the notion that their shame was a source of hidden passion and excitement and could well be an organizer as part of their identity.

It certainly was for Cal. Stemming from his highly eroticized mother–infant dyad, Cal lived proudly in shame all his life. It became his Omnipotent Child. In the group, he avoided all interactions that would lead to an uncovering of his overwhelming grief. As he felt safer with the group, he had a short-lived affair out of town. By arousing the group through his lying and secretiveness, he reenacted his arousal by his mother. His intensely arousing and exciting group interactions concealed the internal conflict over shame, alternating with grief. I pointed out that the most important thing for Cal was arousing and seducing the group. The affair was the only way he felt he could do that. The grief began to emerge as we all understood that his arousal was the profound passionate connection and merger with his sexualized mother. He felt shame in being so intensely involved with his seductive mother and with his constant sexual fantasies. He felt grief over the loss of his intense bond with his mother. He struggled to protect himself from profound grief by repeatedly saying proudly, "No one could live with her and be with her as I can." This construct was his Omnipotent Child. His self-hatred and shame for loving the leader dissipated slowly as he noticed that his grief and longings were a real threat to his Omnipotent Child.

During this phase, the earlier discussion of complaints of the group room shifted to the bad fits with their own bodies and their wishes for different bodies. Issues of obesity, anorexia, bulimia, and excessive weightlifting or exercising were expressed. A woman complained that she never could wear dresses; they just didn't fit her. A patient felt his appetites were too strong, too out of control. Another felt her body was toxic. The excitements of the bodies that don't fit, the appetites that don't fit, became the core of the work.

The Phase of Practicing

The beginning phase of separation–individuation, with its attendant potential anxieties and magical excitements, is referred to as *practicing*. During this period, the anxieties of loss and rapprochement get mixed with a passion that can become loaded with aggression. If so, it brings terror, nightmares, fear of abandonment, and fear of loss of identity. This can lead to inhibitions, shame, and embarrassment. These last affects are derivatives of excitement that have gone awry and become filled with erotic and aggressive energies. This leads to an increased fear of loss of self and of the other person. However, we can see the bursting forth of the discovery of a new self with its capacity for powerful imagination, pleasure, and excitement.

On a coffee table, in my office, there was a hollow papier-mâché duck and a cluster of small cut-glass animal figurines. During the life of one group, the duck was filled with a floral arrangement. A small mouse on the table was removed to another part of the office. Kate was comfortably silent for the first year in the group. She was metaphorically sitting in the therapist's lap to soothe and protect herself from the stimulation of the group. It also allowed her to develop the embryonic beginnings of a new self. Kate suddenly awakened to her fantasy that the duck must have eaten the mouse. She knew it was a fantasy, yet it held important meaning for her, the group, and me. Other groups, in the same room, didn't notice the change at all, but this group, led by Kate's fantasies, was entranced and continued discussing their own fantasies.

Kate followed her fantasy with a dream of Thumbelina dancing on her little fingers. Through the group's excitement with her, Thumbelina eventually became the little girl's clitoris. Much later, the duck that ate the mouse was replaced by the mother who swallowed the enthusiasm and early excitement of the little girl. Later on, after repeated involvement with the group and her new-found imagination, she dreamt that she had given birth to a bag of ice (which was her co-constructed identification with her mother and herself as a cold fish). A live fetus followed the icebag, which was her new, emerging warmth and excitement (Aledort, 2008).

Separation–Individuation

The next phase ushered in the more fully developed experiences of separation and attachment. This required the ability to experience object constancy by remembering, in the mind and in the body, the pleasure and soothing of the other person. If this was in place, this period was filled with the intense pleasure of curiosity about the world and the genitals. Again, if healthy, this period led to new attachments that were based on expectations of pleasure, optimism, and arousal. Regulation was key here: not too much or too little. If this phase was not healthy, then one saw intense castration anxiety, wishes to flee the group, and inchoate anxiety. To some, it felt like a profound loss of identity. Childhood fears of going to school and fears of separating were expressed. The fear of the playground, with its attendant competition and physical activity, was reported, and enacted in the group. Terrifying dreams about loss and abandonment filled the group. Shameful and exciting confessionals about excessive masturbation, and their concomitant fantasies, were efforts to reaffirm that the genitals had not disappeared. The group explored their conflicts around masturbation. The healthy self-identity is organized around optimistic curiosity with expectant regulated pleasure. The Omnipotent Child self-identity is organized around inhibition, a fear of curiosity, a fear of pleasure, and a lack of self-regulation. This "bad fit" passion and excitement was used to stabilize this flawed and damaged identity, thus preventing a healthy exploration of the outside world and internal life.

In a twice weekly group, Edith, who struggled with her appetites all her life, had gastric surgery to control her binge eating and excessive weight gain. Edith was exceptionally successful in negotiating with doctors, and the group, for support to undergo this surgery. She lost 50 pounds; she looked and felt great. She described herself as being at the top of her game. She started to date. She told the group that she was involved with a man who didn't like to use condoms. The group went mad, and a flurry of excitement filled the room. She was puzzled. "What's the problem? You told me I should get laid now." She was without guilt or shame, and the group was perplexed, surprised, and frustrated. This drama continued for at least three sessions, with different variations on the theme. One of the quieter members thought that Edith must be trying to get into the therapist's lap with all this excitement and potential danger she had put herself into. He said it reminded him of when she told the group that she had a similar piece of pottery to one that I had, which made her feel close to me when she looked at it at night. She got sad, and talked of missing the exciting, frustrating attachment to me, and the group, that she had before her weight loss and finding a man. She didn't know how to be intimate and close to us now that she was not so needy, and felt so good. The group was sad. I told Edith that my lap and insides were always open to her. She didn't have to be needy, damaged, or in danger to get in. I explained that I and the other group members could sustain her fullness. It was all right to be in my lap just because it felt good. Using my lap was not being disloyal to her forward strivings nor other positive desires. We warned Edith that her Omnipotent Child would see her growth as disloyal. We alerted her to this internal struggle and helped her as she struggled to maintain her new identity.

Most of the group sustained her full excitement without being threatened. They could tolerate Edith no longer needing them in the way she did before. Cal could not. He wanted her to be fat and needy, so he could feel his self-righteous indignation around her neediness, rather than the excitement of her new-found identity. He wasn't quite ready to deal with his grief at her leaving. Her progress required him to rework his personal Omnipotent Child. Helen was another example from this phase.

Helen came from a family where she was threatened with annihilation throughout most of her childhood. She stayed quiet and hidden. Her Omnipotent Child was labeled as her need to be safe by playing dead in her coffin. Over time, she peeked out from my lap and tried to get involved with others in the group. She was frightened of too much stimulation. She began to see that the passion in her life was to stabilize her life in her magnificently built coffin. In fantasy, the whole group was involved in building the coffin with her. She slowly peeked out, and started to play with the others. She knew she could return to my lap, or my insides, and did many times. Initially I called her back when she got too anxious, but soon she learned to return on her own. Labeling the Omnipotent Child helped unite the group and understand their excitement around each other's Omnipotent Child. It helped externalize the internal, hidden bad fits, and allowed the grandiose shame and humiliation that was attached to the excitement of the bad fit to be broached in the group.

The *witch mother* is always present in this phase, and succeeding ones as well. Her counterpoint is the good mother of rapprochement. As group members struggled to separate, trying to avoid the wrath of the possessive, jealous witch mother, their excitement spilled over to fantasy play. The issue of regulating excitement in the patient and the group, as they wanted to play with each other, was crucial at this stage. They had to contend with the vulnerabilities of too much or too little stimulation and the problem of being precocious. One group played well with each other for a few consecutive sessions. Then one member decided to bring gasoline canisters into the fantasy tree house they had built. The group play imploded to avoid exploding. The heat in the play was premature, and not sufficiently regulated. The Omnipotent Child of unregulated excitement and precocious acting out created the intensely aggressive fantasy play.

Precocious patients get into trouble. Lannie did when she popped her head out too soon and brazenly announced that she could give the therapist an erection by sitting on his lap. Bea did by stating that she was the only fertile woman in the group. Don did by stating that he felt all the women in the group would naturally love and adore him.

The shy patients suffered from shame and envy. They filled the room with tales of shameful episodes in their life. The passion of their shame was sometimes equaled by their hidden envy. Phil became the witch mother when he proudly and humorously talked about his capacity to wring the fun out of any situation with his family and with this group. With this Omnipotent Child, he interfered with their wish to be free and enjoy themselves. Before they could separate from their old bad fits, they needed to reenact the magnificent passion in their bad fits. They all struggled toward a different identity to separate from the excitement of the old bad fit.

These reenactments were possible because of the nature of the analytic culture in the group. This culture allowed the hidden bad fits to be fully expressed and admired before they were given up. It was crucial for the group's progress that these Passionate Bad Fits were seen, in all their glory, heroic loyalty, and wonderment. An appreciation for how important the Omnipotent Child had been to each person was necessary before they could give up the Omnipotent Child.

Al, who was on the spot for provoking the group with his imperious manner, claimed to be a victim. I told him that he was the most provocative person I had worked with in quite a while. A loud belly laugh erupted from him, and the group, as we all joined him in this moment of affective merger with his proud Passionate Bad Fit.

Sexuality, Ambiguity, and Safe Harbors

The group felt unsafe as they became more and more aware of the sexual differences among them. They felt especially vulnerable as they began to form alliances, love relations, and triangles. Passions of competition, envy, and shame were coupled with the joy of discovery. Shame in the group seemed directly related to their struggle toward separation while managing their intense feelings of arousal and dependent longings. Many times, this shame was hidden by the excessive omnipotence of the old bad-fit Omnipotent Child. The group allowed the therapist to come in as the protective parent so that the growth process continued. The group sought attachments that allowed them to practice and cathect newly liberated libidinal and aggressive drives. At the same time, they required someone onto whom they could project the negative introjects that came from their original love object. The depressed, abandoned parent made herself known through a self-selected patient who demanded that the group deal with her depression. For the group to progress, the patient, who was acting as the abandoned mother, must be nurtured by the therapist. Without this, the group would remain stuck.

Other bad-fit passions led to couples banding together to kill off a third person. Bob and Jean went through a three-session giggling phase aimed at killing off Carla, who represented the depressed mother, wrinkling her nose at fun and sexuality.

Jody and Mia, two women who hated men, got together and decided, with great fun and hilarity, that Jody would kill me off and dance on my grave, while Mia would defend her in court on the murder charges. Both women, at this time, were asexual. The other pairing was of the "sob sisters," who joined each other in their mutual disappointment in men and sexuality.

The fantasy power of the therapist/father entered the room in different forms. Fantasies of love and hate dominated, as well as fantasies of how babies were born. There was much curiosity about the parental bedroom. I encouraged and contained the anxieties about these issues. Many times they were expressed through their erotic dreams, excitement, and corresponding shameful feelings and surprises.

Howie, who lived in the shame of being controlled by his wife, struggled to tell Robin he liked her very much. He found her attractive, but was ashamed to say anything because he wished she would wear different glasses. He struggled with the group as to what was more exciting, the shame of wanting to ask, or the pleasure of getting closer to Robin. If he asked her, he was taking a risk. The risk was opening a new door into the passionate good fit. The shame and the excitement co-existed. The real danger, as opposed to the safe harbor, was the patients' needs to treasure the negative introjects and to worship them. The group's Omnipotent Child and individual member's Omnipotent Child inhibited healthy fantasies and connections.

The next phase, the working-through phase, was ushered in by intense curiosity about learning how to master strong desires. The group now made more demands on each other without shame and anxiety. The good mother of rapprochement was more available to soothe when arousal and pleasure turned to fear and dread. When this happened, the excitement in the body was not seen as an enemy, but as an ally. Bigness, and how it affected dreams and fantasies, came to the fore.

A twice-weekly group arrived at this advanced stage and noticed that few dreams were coming into the group. They were curious about why this was happening. Amy, a sexy, attractive young woman had just joined the group. Two people talked about never remembering their dreams. Dinah reported going to a business conference where she did well and, in her exuberance, tripped all over herself. The group and I wondered if perhaps she was trying to fly. The group was asked to imagine what it would be like to fly and be big. Dinah stammered and then smiled seductively toward me. She was asked to think of the biggest fantasy she could have, perhaps wanting to have me all for herself. The group laughed and said I was incorrigible. Dinah related her sexualized associations to floats at the Macy's Thanksgiving Day Parade. Paul chimed in with the Woody Woodpecker float from Seinfeld. The group laughed uneasily. Paul recalled a dream about being friendly to a big elephant. I said Paul was trying to be close to his own bigness, sexuality, and fantasies. At the next session, the group continued to hear stories about Paul's wife's discomfort with her sexual fantasies toward him. The new member was upset with her friend's sexual acting out at her business meeting. The group was able to connect their fear of remembering their dreams and the fantasies that had emerged recently, with their discomfort in their healthy state of bigness. They recognized that they were frightened of where it would take them in the group. During this phase, the excitement of trying on a new identity, and speaking the unspeakable, became the organizers of the group activity.

The Working–through Phase

This was the working-through phase of the Passionate Bad Fits. Critical to this phase was being able to be aware of the excitement of the passion that was in the good fit. And, even though it may not have that same rush and intense somatic sensation as in the bad fits, it is real and alive. We all have experienced the patient who finds a good nurturing woman or man but just doesn't find the sexual excitement present. Howie struggled with his new-found independence after leaving his wife of 25 years. For 18 years they had no sex. Though he pursued sexy women, he re-created his empty marriage. The women treated him just as badly as his wife did. He defended against this mistreatment by being excessively understanding and compassionate to them. He was their good therapist and savior. He and the group were dismayed when the therapist pointed out his longstanding, and only recently discovered, Omnipotent Child, of being the most compassionate man who didn't notice how badly he was treated.

The loss and mourning over the Omnipotent Child was the shared excitement in this phase. Now, the dreaded anxiety of establishing a new identity was one of the most powerful affective experiences. Judy was agonized when she realized that she had to separate from her Omnipotent Child. The Omnipotent Child was too costly, and she was filled with rage and sadness over the many regrets she had about her life. She dreamt of falling into a canyon, had nightmares of losing herself, got into impasse struggles with the therapist, and was terrified for weeks. She had lost her best friend; she cried, and felt like something was stirring inside of her that felt nameless. The new Judy and the group survived. The group held Judy and helped her to contain the anxiety she felt over her enormous loss.

The excitement of leaving the group, of finding someone new in their lives, as well as a new respect for themselves, fortified the group culture. Patients felt less corrupt; they felt they could tolerate envy, and enjoy each other's successes. There was excitement from the senior members as they welcomed new members into the group. They shared their acquired wisdom. There was excitement as they told of loving someone, being loved, and truly missing people in the group. The group experienced powerful moments when they took each other in, let each other inside, and metaphorically sat on each other's laps. These mutual mergers solidified the new embryonic good fits and the new identities. The group could cry together as some members left and new ones entered.

Conclusion

When one focuses on the excitement and passion attached to the bad fits, new avenues of thinking, insight, and interpretation open for the therapist and the group. The issue of resistance is seen differently. Resistant behaviors are seen as the effort to preserve the excitement of the old, bad fits. Resistance is now connected to the relinquishing of the Omnipotent Child in the different developmental phases of the work. Until the passion holding this is analyzed, the patient cannot enjoy healthier templates of intimacy and thus a healthier identity.

The group is the perfect setting for the re-enactments of the old bad fits. If one allows the bad fits to be expanded and adored, put into perspective of their origin, shame begins to dwindle. One is then more able to help patients move toward an empathetic awareness of the power of the earliest bad fits in their life. Moments of merger experienced in the group afford opportunities to analyze the excitement in these highly somatic, affective experiences. As patients mourn their early fate and appreciate the power of the passion of the bad fit, adult choices seem more possible.

Note

1 Reprinted from *GROUP*, Vol. 33, No.1, pp. 45–63, March 2009. Used with permission.

Chapter 18

Sexuality in Group

Sexuality is a developmental process. As such, it needs to be attended to, along with other developmental tasks. The group process is ideal for the working through of sexual issues. The therapist must be ever-present, from the inception of the group until it ends. Nitsun (2006) says the therapist is an active presence in the group. As we know, the therapist has a considerable impact on the group. Most therapists are reluctant to address these issues, partly because there has been very little training for them, and also because of a lack of comfort in their own sexuality. How comfortable are therapists with being the objects of desire and being aware and working with their desire toward their patients, especially in groups? Are therapists trained in understanding the significance of analyzing and working with sexual fantasies and actions in their groups and in themselves? Are therapists trained to differentiate eroticized conflicts, versus countertransference and real sexual feelings? Can they rely on their capacity to have mastery over their own feelings?

In my model, the construct of the Omnipotent Child and its developmental underlying structure, i.e., the Passionate Bad Fit, come to the fore and are examined through the relationships in the group. The construct of the Omnipotent Child describes the psychological residues of bad fits that occur during development when the psychological states of the mothering figure do not attune with the child's developing needs. These experiences become core identity elements and affect the templates of intimacy in all future relationships. This Omnipotent Child is quite powerful and prevents healthier attachments in a person's life. The work in this model promotes separations from these old bad fits and creation of newer, different attachments. These newer attachments are perceived by the group as less passionate and therefore less desirable. Sexuality in its myriad forms clearly fits into the potential for Passionate Bad Fits.

Sexuality is a highly charged somatic affect, whether in fantasy or reality, that has enormous influence on core identity and templates of intimacy. Therefore, sexuality has to be worked with in each developmental phase. I will refer now to the different phases that the group goes through to evolve into a relatively healthy adult with a good relationship to his body, the body as ally, not enemy, as well as a healthy relationship with his fantasy life and with his sexual desires.

DOI: 10.4324/9781032705835-22

Walter, a 67-year-old man who recently came into the group, described a 40-year struggle with depression. As we learned, he and his mother had a remarkable love relationship. In the group, we were able to help him see that his struggle was with his idea that desire would either lead to incest or homosexuality. The issue we are addressing is his needing to feel safe with the group in a state of desire, whether he is homosexual or not. His Omnipotent Child was organized around how he can endure a life without desire. How sad it has been for him to do without desire most of his adult life.

Phase I: The Fit, the Lap, and the Symbiotic Mother

In the opening phase, as the therapist demands the group come to him as the mother of symbiosis, the room becomes the pre-verbal dyad body in various states of attunement or misattunement. The room can never be quite right. It is too dark, too light, too noisy, too silent, too stimulating, or not stimulating enough. The sexuality in this pre-verbal phase is in the bodily experience of trying to regulate the degree of stimulation. Some members will view my invitation to the lap as a sexual seduction from the father. The therapist must know and have mastery over, his own boundaries and desires. Premature sexuality is always ready to rear its head. The concurrent theme and mental experience in this phase is the fantasy of being inside the object of desire, which predates the later experience of intercourse, merger, and romantic excitement in the somatic closeness. The issue of safety, and what the therapist can contain and deal with, is critical.

The therapist has to be acutely aware of his level of excitement, and potential over-stimulation or withdrawal from this provocative relationship. To promote the growth of the mother–infant or group–individual dyad, the bigness of the therapist must be present and acknowledged.

The importance of regulating the therapist's bigness, excitement, self-centeredness, and responsibility is similar to the passion of the mother regulating her self-centeredness, anxieties, excitements, and pleasures, and her need to meet the corresponding regulation of the infant's needs. Fonagy (1999) stated that co-regulation was defined as behavior that was unfolding in an individual while simultaneously being modified by the changing behavior of a partner. These processes were mostly preverbal, like Ashley and her silence, and the excitement of being with a good mother who makes no demands on her, other than letting her be in our arms as long she wishes to be. I am constantly checking if this is still all right with her, as her whole life is changing dramatically. These passionate moments lead to sustaining the co-regulation, which is imperative in the development of a strong healthy life of excitement and sexuality.

Phase II: Separation and Individuation

The next developmental phase is the beginning of hatching and practicing in the separation–individuation continuum. The task for the group is the exploration of the magical thinking of early childhood, which expresses the surprise and wonderment at both the separation from the symbiotic mother and discovery of their own genitals. The group must now learn to look at each other with intense curiosity and excitement but without action and panic. They want to know if it is all right to be excited by their discoveries, both in their bodies and in their thoughts and dreams.

The group is filled with the excitement of giggling, dreams, storytelling, jokes, and people asking personal questions of themselves and others. The emergence of a group historian, recorder, and timekeeper keeps the group from regressing back to the symbiotic mother. This phase charges the body and mind to the aspect of relationships as little kids. Early falling in love can take place here. Awe and wonderment in the other at times can fill the room.

> Tom couldn't help but look at Mary and feel wonderful and excited and full. But he was so easily injured when Mary didn't return his ardor, so he returned to the lap for comfort. Tom loved to be in awe and Mary loved to reject. The playground can be dangerous, exciting and wonderful. The group's reveling in the injuries in the playground in the passionate bad fit gets exposed. Precocious sexuality occurs here, as does excessive aggression.
>
> One group, engaged in fantasy play, was doing well until Beth decided to bring kerosene to the playhouse and set fire to it. Her heat and rage at being left out later became the origin for her inability to accept how important she was to the group, even though she was the biggest critic and lacked the most empathy for others in the group. She decided to make love to me and forget the kids in the playground. She was quite specific about how she was going to sit on me and screw the living daylights out of me. She said that I would never have a better lover. I said, "That could be, but it tells us how exciting your precociousness must be to you and how it gets you into trouble with the other kids. You need to be in my lap, not screwing me."

Phase III: Sexuality, Ambiguity, and Safe Harbors

The therapist's role is to help facilitate dreams, fantasies, and object attachments while ensuring a safe harbor from the enraged, abandoned pre-oedipal parent or the over-stimulated parent. The group is excited and stimulated by the sexual differences and their own histories about their knowing.

> Paul proclaimed incessantly that he would never be excited by the group and thoroughly enjoyed squelching the others' excitements. Eva and Myrna bonded together as sisters wedded to the destruction of men. Their bond was filled with homoerotic fantasies and underlying was their Omnipotent Child of never surrendering to a man. Coupling was promoted by me, and Harry and Alice in particular struggled with my comments about their mutual involvement. Harry struggled with intensely sexual fantasies of his mother, in the face of a passive father. Alice struggled with her lust for a gay friend and her intense

discomfort at exposing her excitement in her life and in the group. They had dreams of each other. Alice could not work with my being the object of her sexual thoughts, but Harry then moved in with his dreams and fantasies of his eroticized relationship with his mother. The foundation for the classical triangle was being structured.

The narcissistic issues in this phase are the grandiose fantasies of having and owning the only true genital. The notion of women as castrated men, the fantasy of the phallic women, the power of the female genitals, and anxiety over penis and womb envy become focal points for the Omnipotent Child in this phase, and clearly represent earlier Passionate Bad Fits in these body images. These bad fits tend to diffuse the intense longing and concomitant surrender to the other.

A sign that the excitement in the group is over-stimulating, or filled with too much conflict about desire, can be noted if a member finds a boyfriend or lover shortly after joining the group.

Resa, 41, technically still a virgin, holds on to her need to see men as her father. To counter her seeing me as a jackass, i.e., like her father, she quickly got involved with her boss in a father–daughter mutually seductive but frustrating alliance. She feels she needs this until she can feel safe with a man. Buddy plays along with this by seeing her and calling her Baby Resa. Buddy, who is suffused with sexual fantasies from earlier experiences of seduction by his mother, has to sap the sexuality out of all the women in the group, at the same time stimulating them with his tales of sexual preoccupations, including an affair with an out-of-town woman he lied about and then acknowledged to the group. Sometimes the sexuality gets embedded in one patient. That can potentially lead to an early departure from the group.

Brenda lives in the Omnipotent Child of the inadequate, failed woman. She begins to change her identity while in fantasy on my lap and inside of me. She feels that she is in the inside of a different mother, who lets her know that she will be encouraged to be excited, sexual, and not depressed. She lets a strong woman in the group help her to have a makeover—different hairdo, different clothes, etc. She then falls madly in love with Mel. Unlike Resa, she lets the group teach her about her own body and how to enjoy and masturbate for the first time. Mel, who is still recovering from being fused with a psychotic, seductive mother, smiled with delight that Brenda would like him. He felt safe with her and was able in fantasy to join her on the floor as she experienced what sex with him would be like. He said that this experience kept him separate, less afraid and not fused, and still passionately connected to her. He still would like to live by himself, but he didn't feel as alone. The sexuality and fantasies serve as a bridge to both expose their Omnipotent Children and attempt to try out different experiences within the framework of the group as they realized that they now have begun the process of changing their internal perceptions of themselves.

Phase IV: The Analytic Culture

This phase represents the work of separating from the Omnipotent Child by developing and luxuriating in the Passionate Good Fit, which is the only antidote to the Passionate Bad Fit. Reworked relationships, new relationships, new excitements, new chances and risks, and exposure of shameful conflicts have to be resolved and experienced.

> Buddy is both hypersexual and terrified of his desire to merge with the woman. This stems from his early bad fit with an over-stimulating mother. Harry has his intense sexual desires for mother transferred to his aunt and all other women save for his wife. His Omnipotent Child was his fear of his sexuality and aggression, while at the same time being flooded with sexual fantasies. Gloria acts like a sexual vamp in the group as a defense against talking about her shame from her sexually abusive background. Following her divorce, she got sexually involved with a younger, sadistic man, who put her in constant danger and shame. Alice. who has been married twice, is now entangled in a frustrating, arousing relationship with a gay male co-worker. She is unable to relate to me in a desiring way, but has found Harry, and Harry has found the sexy mother in the group. Resa had a father who was hypersexual, with multiple affairs and aggression that frightened her away from having normal oedipal feelings. For safety, she's involved in an intense loving but restricted sexual relationship with her boss. This way she avoids me as the stimulating father in the group. Buddy sees her as baby Resa to protect himself from her sexuality and from his rage at women. He conspires to get rid of a highly sexy young woman, Molly, by telling her that the group talked behind her back about her sexual promiscuity. Molly left the group shortly thereafter. Myrna, who is in a termination phase with the group, is in a very mature relationship with a man I see in individual therapy who she had to tame from his intense S&M fantasies and activities with her. She deals with her feelings toward me by reliving over and over her disappointments with me in the work. We both can now appreciate how exciting and arousing her diatribes toward me are. She needs to conceal the sexiness to protect against the enraged depressed mother lurking in the group. She is now appreciating her yearnings and warm feelings toward me and our mutual deep caring for each other, without the fear of losing her good mother. She is less shocked now when the group wants her contribute more often.
>   The group periodically, and more now, gets into sexually exciting experiences. Buddy usually starts it. The recent go-around started with the issue of Buddy not having oral sex with his wife. The group was incredulous since he has daily sexual fantasies about any woman he sees. This led to a round of exciting laughter and shameful moments of silence, and then a discussion of the woman's genitals and what to do with them and how the women loved to have oral sex and the men agreeing and then Resa wanted to know what the vagina looked like. She is getting ready to be fully sexual with a boyfriend in another

state. When the group bogged down, I wondered aloud if it got bogged down on the clitoris. This was met with a great round of laughter and anxiety. The group felt close, people told Resa to read *Our Body Ourselves*. Gloria was surprised that we could all connect this way, and Alice felt more alive than she had let herself be in ages. Of course, the next session was dull and the group could see the function of their resistance or their need to take a timeout and regulate the excitement in the new exciting safe play. The moments of excitement and arousal were with all of us now and it picked up again after another session. As we talked and experienced sexual excitement. the usual lateness in this group had disappeared. They were ready to go when I opened the door to the group room.

Chapter 19

Sitting in the Hot Seat[1]

Dilemma: Tolerating the Intolerable

I have been running a psychodynamic group for 15 years with varying membership over that time. The group consists of four men and four women, all of whom are in their late 30s to mid-50s and are professionals or in the arts. My group is a lively one, with lots of intelligent conversation, banter, and good will among the members. The members can also go deep with each other. They have dealt with the death of a child, failed marriages, empty nests, family illness, new spouses, graduations, and taking care of elderly parents. They have been able to deal with conflict so well, I sometimes wonder if I am even needed. Recently two members really had it out with each other, yet they were able to work out the conflict without yelling, leaving, or shaming each other. I am impressed and sometimes awed by how well the group works together and by the members' level of attachment, which brings me to the following dilemma.

Sometimes I feel like I am the least well-functioning person in the room, even though I am happily married and have two young children at home. Life hadn't been easy, and, like many therapists, I had a rough childhood, but I spent a lot of years in therapy working out my issues. I'm also in supervision, which helps me metabolize my feelings. However, recently I have found myself attracted to a particular man in the group and have had a hard time managing my feelings. He is a bit of a flirt, and I feel like a teenager who is smitten. Claudio is Italian, intelligent, handsome, funny, warm, and newly married to a woman he met online. He is here in the States for several years as a researcher in biotech, working on serious cancer drugs while his wife remains in Italy with the children. When he talks of his teenagers, he does so with such love and caring that I yearn for him to be part of my family. I find myself dreaming about him and become jealous when he shows attention to the women in the group. I know these feelings are normal to have when one works closely with patients, but I am finding it difficult to hide how I feel in the group. Recently, he teased me with a minor sexual innuendo, and I felt myself blush. The group noticed and laughed, but I felt exposed. The group seems to like his humor and flirting, and many of the women, and even the men, flirt with him. They don't seem to feel threatened by him the way I do.

DOI: 10.4324/9781032705835-23

While I know I will not act on my feelings, I feel nervous when I am running the group. I have not found a way to address his flirting in the group, because I am afraid my feelings will show. I have stopped addressing him directly (I'll ask someone else what they think is going on with him), and I avoid his gaze. I also have become hypervigilant about boundaries, addressing every minor infraction from being one minute late to not paying the bill. I also wondered aloud about the playful quality of the group and whether the group is avoiding something deeper. While I have always addressed boundary issues in the group before, I feel that I have begun to nitpick the group as a way of managing my own sexual feelings.

Lately, I have begun to wonder why my feelings are so intense and whether there is something also going on in the group that I am unaware of. I fantasize that two members may be having an affair, or that group members are meeting outside the group. I have also had experiences in the past where I have "hated" a patient or felt motherly toward one. And I've often felt like I want to be part of a group that I am running. But the feelings I have described above have lasted the longest and feel draining. Can you help me better understand what might be going on in the group? Do other people feel this intensely?

Up to this point, this group has clearly done extremely well. It is quite mature in dealing with life issues. I really can empathize with your dilemma. In running my long-term groups, I've been there many times and have learned an enormous amount from these dilemmas. I hope I can help you with yours. My orientation is psychoanalytic. I've been heavily influenced by Margaret Mahler's (1968) developmental model and Kohut's (1978) exploration of grandiosity and the narcissistic lines of development. I'm particularly focused on the role of pre-verbal experiences and the passion in both the good and bad fits. My theoretical construct is that the earliest misattunements are experienced somatically in the dyad, and these moments lay down neuronal pathways in the right hemisphere. These can then become that part of the body ego that contains the Passionate Bad Fits. I have called this part the *Omnipotent Child* that has now morphed into the Passionate Bad Fits. These Passionate Bad Fits not only tell the early story but also have enormous influence on the patient's templates of intimacy and identity. The need to keep the bad-fit identity intact is profound. As such, it is the source of the repetitive re-enactments in the group and in members' lives. To do this work, the group culture develops by the leader assuming the mantle of the mother of symbiosis (Mahler, 1968), and patients, at the beginning, are experienced as infants trying to recreate and/or tell their stories of the preverbal experiences in their lives. The telling of the stories usually precedes and sets up the ensuing re-enactments. This crucial work can be done at the beginning of the group in the first year or two, which is my preference, but if it isn't then it demands to be done later. This dilemma suggests that is what is going on in the group now.

There have been many times when I too wished to be a member of the group that I run. But why? I assume that all therapists have difficult issues to work on in their lives. I think we are all vulnerable to regress to the state of wordless bliss that Mahler (1968) calls the *autistic phase*. To be one with the group is delicious, exciting, and passionate, but doesn't allow us to notice deeper issues that are going on with ourselves and with the group. I think that your romance with Claudio is a good example of this blissful state that you would like to attain, but in the blissful romance, you have lost a part of your identity as therapist.

You are now faced with holding the very difficult feelings of shame and desire. I have written recently on shame and the hidden excitement that keeps it alive. Shame is a primary affect and can be seen in the early preverbal dyad (Alonso & Rutan, 1988). I have postulated that the early shameful feelings are intensified by the somatic Passionate Bad Fits in this early pre-verbal life. I'm talking about shame now because I really believe it's an answer to the question that you raise, which is that you think there's something deeper going on in the group. You are right. There is for all of you.

You have let me know of hidden sexual feelings toward Claudio. But now in your fantasy life, they have extended to hidden sexual acting out within the group. The first clue that locates the problem to passionate shame in the early preverbal period in life is your acute awareness of your own internal conflicts and your struggles to put them into words. When a therapist can't find words, I assume that she is re-experiencing for herself (or the group) a pre-verbal period of life. She also shows some signs of shame, with its attendant somatic blushing and fearful glances. While you are in a painful fantasy wish for an erotic, blissful cocoon with Claudio, the group is playing out their shameless, grandiose excitement through flirting, teasing each other, and dismissing the therapist. You are in pain while the group is painlessly excited. You are carrying the shame and hidden excitement for the group. The group is playing out the excitement in your shame. At the same time, you feel you have to hide your exciting romantic and erotic feelings toward Claudio and are very concerned about exposing your feelings. Blushing is one of the somatic exciting experiences in shame. I'm also struck with how you talked about all the different issues that this mature group has worked through. However, there is really no mention of shame. In fact, you talked about how there was an intense conflict between two members and they resolved it without shaming each other.

So I have to ask both of us, why shame now? Why does this become an important component of the group that you are holding? I would love to know the content of the fight between the two members of the group. The content of this fight may throw some light on the hidden feelings in all of you. Is it easier for you and the group that the men fight as a way not to notice the hidden re-enactments of shame and desire? My assumption is that this mature group did not deal with the early hidden exciting shameful feelings in the group, as well as in their own lives in their early preverbal experiences. This group, after five years of secure bonding attachments, affiliation, and working through together, are now more capable and more willing to look at the early preverbal experiences of injury, shame, and excitement. From my work with intensive groups over the years, I have found that when the early preverbal experiences are not dealt with in depth and re-enactment in the group, they make a demand on the group and on the therapist to deal with them, sooner or later. I would also suggest, as the group has, to look at why they need to deal with shame. You would need to look closely at whether, at this time in your personal life, with two young kids, you need to be refueled. You silenced yourself, as I mentioned earlier, possibly as a way not to expose the group to your neediness and object hunger as the little girl demanding a good mother. Doing this work, being the good mother, is always tiring for the therapist. When do we get our turn? So, in terms of your question: Is something going on in the group? My feeling is firmly, yes. And there is something going on in you.

The group, as you describe it, seems to me as if they are a group of early adolescents thoroughly enjoying their eroticism, their flirtatiousness, their excitement, and desires. At the same time, they are rendering you impotent and ineffectual, and most likely enjoying putting you on the spot and making you feel ashamed. You feel they are acting out around payment and coming on time. You should be suspicious of the playful group. The play of the group, I'm afraid, is at your expense and theirs. Your "nitpicking" the group is not just a result of your attempt to manage your own sexual feelings but is also a way to reestablish your identity as the group therapist. To further reestablish your identity, we have to deal with the Claudio issue. What to say and how to say it? These are the moments that make the work so magnificent. How much to disclose and what should be disclosed? What is the goal of self-disclosure? Should there be any self-disclosure at this point? In my theoretical framework, the therapist is crucial in all phases of the group. The buck stops at the therapist's door. You must free yourself of the projected introjects of hidden shame, as well as your vulnerability to your exciting shameful fantasies. You first have to get comfortable with the intensity of these powerful fantasies by seeing them as a means to help the group explore their shameful and exciting fantasies. You let me know that you are vulnerable to strong affects that arise in the group, and in particular to your investment in some individual patients in the group, like the ones you "hate or want to mother." This is your most valuable asset in doing this complex work. What is crucial is how we work with these strong affects.

When the shame shows, I believe it is important to give the group a reality check. It also serves as a model to let the group know about the hidden excitement that keeps shame alive. If you hold on to it, you then can intensify any vulnerabilities that stabilize a bad fit identity with shame as an organizer. In this instance, I might say something like this:

> I notice that the group is very involved with flirting with and admiring Claudio. I too find Claudio a very exciting man. I'm sure all of you have noticed that I blush about these feelings and that it's hard for me to speak directly with Claudio. I know that these are symptoms and expressions of shame. It seems to me that maybe the group really hasn't spent enough time talking about hidden shame in their current lives, in the group with me, and in their early lives. What do people

know about shame in their lives? What was it like for Claudio to be the object of desire in his early life? What is it like for the group to try to render me impotent?

I think these kinds of comments can restore you to your desired role as an active, meaningful therapist, and will also give the group a chance to talk about how they dismissed their own parents or rendered them incompetent. I think you have held the more dangerous aspects of adolescent flirtations and grandiose behavior. It feels like envy is in the room but you are holding it to protect them and yourself from owning aggressive and rivalrous feelings.

Early in my career, I didn't pay much attention to shame in the group. Shame felt too overwhelming to deal with, and it also felt too personal, and no one ever talked about or taught me how to deal with shame. I would never reveal anything personal about how I felt, since I was trained in the classical psychoanalytic model of the blank screen. I am now much more comfortable working with and trying to flesh out shame in groups I run, as well as disclosing how I feel about what's happening in the room. I still disclose almost nothing about my personal life, like where I'm going on vacation, my children, etc. I have, however, filled my room with objects of my life that clearly disclose who I am. I also believe that, as part of the centrality of the therapist's role in all phases of development, the therapist must lend him- or herself to become the object of desire, whatever the desire is. Are you comfortable being the object of the group's desire, or are you enabling Claudio to rescue you from that role? As you can see, your fears, anxieties, and fantasies really open up so many avenues of exploration for the group. They can go back and talk about the exciting desires in their early years. This will be instrumental to developing further growth in this group, and your own growth.

One can also see this dilemma as the group's step toward further mutual growth and further separation and individuation from the therapist. The therapist's fantasies toward Claudio could be seen as her way of holding on to the group before acknowledging that they have to leave or that they don't need her as much as they used to. She feels badly about not wanting them to leave and then punishes herself. In this vein, the therapist may say, "I've noticed that the group seems to be relying less on me all the time and I wonder what that feels like to the group at this point in our work together." The concepts of desire, excitement, and shame would not be in the therapist's mind. Her focus would be mainly on separation–individuation and loss.

Relational analysts would try to focus on the co-creation between the group and the therapist to help transform re-enactments into corrective emotional experiences in the here and now in the group. They would postulate that the therapist and Claudio are re-enacting their earlier lives of possibly too much stimulation in the mother–child dyad. This may have led to intense arousing fantasies in both of them that could lead to shame and acting out. The comments the relational therapist might make would require more self-disclosure than I am personally comfortable with. You would have to make your choices about that. You might say,

I've noticed that I've been filled with shameful sexual fantasies and helpless feelings about being your therapist and not being needed. I'm wondering if these internal feelings reflect periods of overstimulation that the group has experienced that may have led to shameful desires and acting out, and feelings of helplessness to control them.

There are many options to deal with this dilemma. I have tried to present the one that has worked for me over time. You need to find a way to deal with interpersonal and intrapsychic shame to complement the makings of a fine group therapist.

Note

1 Reprinted from *Complex Dilemmas in Group Therapy: Pathways to Resolution,* second edition, L Motherwell & J. Shay, Eds., pp. 135–138. © 2014 by Routledge. Reproduced by permission of Taylor & Francis Group.

Part V

Retirement
The Final Chapter

Chapter 20

Retiring after over 50 Years in Practice

Part One

How can one do that without getting mired in a complex series of feelings, fantasies, conflicts, conscious and unconscious moments, dreams, and all the rest that humanity has to offer? I experienced all of those things, and still do, as I write this for my book, for me, and for my groups. I have run three once-weekly intensive psychotherapy groups for the last 50 years here in Washington DC. I have run three professional training groups for the last 30 years that meet semi-annually for a full weekend experience, two located in Washington, DC, and one in New York. I love my groups—they sustain me—and I always have had the wish that I could be a member of one of my groups—the ultimate in narcissistic wishes.

For the last year or two, I have played with the notion of retiring. I am 84 at this writing. The first thoughts of retirement were filled with pleasure, traveling with my wife, friends, family, and continuing in our state of joy forever. We talked about both of us going at the same time. We laughed as we looked death in the face, as in a Bergman movie. We would always cry and hug after knowing that neither of us would ever leave the other.

In my language, we were joined in the mutual grandiosity that everyone keeps longing for to heal the abrupt rupture of their moments of grandiosity at birth. The rupture leaves an enormous number of people in constant melancholy, grief, outrage, and helplessness to keep searching and to survive the loss and disillusionment. Our vows did not work, and she died rather quickly two years ago (2020) from a highly malignant lung cancer. I was devastated, scared, terrified about being alone, and lost in the valley of needing a new identity to sustain me and let me go on working with my patients. Life itself felt like it took a back seat to my work. I needed my groups to sustain me and therefore walked a very slippery slope so as to not act that out with them. In the past, I tended to be very harsh with therapists who disclosed too much. I thought they gave up their role of the therapist and became one of the patients. To my surprise, now I wanted to tell all. I wanted my groups to become my beloved Sheila. I wanted the groups to embrace me and never let me go. I wanted and needed to be adored by them, to take over my life decisions, and to still hold my head up and feel like I was a good therapist.

DOI: 10.4324/9781032705835-25

Since then, I have had to make major adjustments to my lifestyle, from my beautiful house in Georgetown with all the help we needed, the friends we loved, and the families close by. It was ideal, and the marriage was just the way it should be. I ended up in a very lovely residential center living by myself in the middle of DC—a place that my spouse did not like at all and never would have come to with me, if that situation had developed. I had to grow up quickly, and I was a very unhappy camper. Who was I without a woman to lean on, to expect her to know me better than I know myself, a woman who had all the answers, and would shape me, at times control me, and feed me, and at the same time let me be autonomous and able to do what I wanted to do without shame and guilt?

My wife, Sheila, spurred me on to let the AGPA and my other peers know how I run groups and the theory behind it. I never imagined that I could be a theoretician and actually create out of my experiences, studies, and training a new theory that embodied not only who I was but also what my patients were telling me. They were all saying they needed more. They almost all had previous therapy, yet fundamentally they felt they stayed the same. I had that feeling from my own analysis, when my analyst asked me as I was ending the analysis what I had gained. I took a deep breath and said that I came in troubled that I could not swallow any medication that I needed. I said that I can now swallow my pills; if I could swallow you and how you practice analysis, I guess I could swallow my pills. I was always the rebel and will most likely continue until I die.

Sheila was my editor, persuader, and fierce rooter for taking myself more seriously than I did. She was right. I never took myself seriously as an excellent therapist who could develop an alternate theory and technique in psychoanalytic group therapy. I stood tall. I still stand tall today, but I feel like a different person now. I really feel that I like myself better.

I have been trying to live in my Passionate Good Fit for the last year and a half. I wondered whether the Passionate Good Fit of my marriage would translate to my new life. It did, with some different internal changes as well. I no longer fear being alone. At times, I crave it and now see it as a crucial part of life that needs to be taken seriously. I began to notice that, as I explored on my own, my therapy work began to shift, and my ability to write and try this book seemed reasonable. I had to redefine myself without my Sheila.

What did I do with my acute grief as I worked with my groups? I tended to reveal very little of my life to my patients. My office is filled with people and artifacts of my life, but my personal life was mine and not theirs. That is how I worked all these years.

After her death, I could not keep working without sharing my loss with the group. My state of mind and affect demanded it, even though they were curious at my unexpected absence from the group for two weeks. They were relieved and saddened by what I told them. I went on a reading spree to learn as much as I could about death and recovery. I reread Yalom's (2021) book on death and life. I plunged into Oliver Sacks's (1983, 1993, 2007) writings about the human condition and how we all attempt to adapt to our internal bio-neuronal system. I read Malcolm (1981), Mitchell (1993), and Frankl (1984), and an article about the death of a group therapist (Rice, Shapiro, & Shay, 2011).

What is grief? It allowed me to really cry for the first time since my older brother's death. It felt relieving to sob and feel her loss and my fear and terror about what parts of me would remain that I will recognize. I was not sure, but the groups were a piece of grounded reality for me that stabilized the grief, and made it feel more real and more mine. I was without shame and guilt, as I began to recognize. I was proud of my grief. It let the world know how lucky I was to have found my Sheila. I had plenty of tryouts, but this one landed me in the big leagues. I felt like Jackie Robinson must have felt as a Brooklyn Dodger. I belonged in the grieving circles, and yet so lucky at being able to grieve that lost love.

My dear close friends comforted me, understood my grief, let me talk, and shared memories together of Sheila and me as a couple. I believed that the groups could handle what I was telling them. I really got a sense of the magnitude of enjoying healthy narcissism, in the face of loss and fear, and how I wanted my groups to try to feel those moments of healthy narcissism without shame. It felt to me that I had to share with them my loss, as my emotions refused to stay hidden. I was disclosing but believed that it was in support of their losses, their shame around the losses, their difficulty in recovering, and, most importantly, their earliest loss of grandiosity shortly after birth. Of course, they did not remember those moments, but their bodies held those memories.

I shared with the groups that my search to recapture my own grandiosity would never help me adjust and grow in the rest of my life. Some in my New York training group knew me and Sheila as a couple, while the Washington groups did not. They asked questions and I told them she was the love of my life, and how bereft I was. I told them that I would be here for them for as long as I can do it, and that I am trying to take good care of myself. I would report any change in that scenario if and when it came up. (I made a slightly different disclosure to the three groups in DC.)

I thought that this could be seen as a model of healthy narcissism without shame and guilt. The group members' responses over time echoed that feeling in them. They were shocked at the disclosure but relieved that I could trust them enough to share this with them. They talked about how they knew very little of their parents' insides. What a relief they felt. "Do you mean that we don't have to take care of you?" they said in three different groups. Could they be and say whatever they wanted now? Could I still be their wonderful therapist who they love, argue with, and are puzzled or angered by what I give them?

They were all shocked that this was the same guy who could take anything they threw at him. Am I the same therapist that seemed to love his work and his passion and expected us to search for that for ourselves? I used my passion for my spouse as a good fit, versus the unconscious passion of the bad fit that bubbles in all of us, leading us to lament our loss and live like a personal injury has been done to us. "How can you do this to me?" filled with self-righteous indignation. I live the despair of victimhood and fill myself with thoughts that tend to negate how my grief showed me the intensity of how I lived and loved with Sheila.

There were members of the group who felt I had come back too soon, that I was not taking good enough care of myself. Their parents, they felt, never took the good care of themselves. They really did not know how to take care of themselves. How can you live with that loss? They could not, they said. I said I was struck that the groups were not talking about their own deep losses, and there were many in the group. There were the losses of mothers, fathers, siblings, and marriages. Also, there were the losses of dreams, ideals, fantasies, hope, healthy body images, and, most importantly, the loss of self-respect as they were beginning to really get into the journey of trying out living in the world of their Passionate Good Fit.

At this point in the group's growth, there is a need to try to define and see clearly their own Omnipotent Child and how they are reliving their older Passionate Bad Fit in the group, and in their life outside. They, with my help, begin to understand how they managed to stay close to the parent that was most difficult to love. They would merge with the most difficult part of that parent, and call it love. But now the parent is inside them, and the imagined closeness hides the toxicity of this merger. The merger is the search for the recapture of the lost omnipotence. The merger recaptures it, with the parent's shame underlying the grandiosity.

Shame is the culprit. Shame is the residue of the ruptures in early life and future hurts. Shame is powerful, is erotic, demands to be part of the internal psyche, and keeps you in a magnificent Passionate Bad Fit. Shame represents failure that becomes magnificent and worshipful. It is the energy and the source of the power of the Omnipotent Child. It has also remained hidden in the psychoanalytic literature, as well as the group literature, and is allowed to go unanalyzed and not seen as one of the strongest drives. There is a need to stay merged and stay close to the object of our hurt (and at times disgust), to live in shame, to keep it hidden, and to romanticize it. There is nothing, it has been reported many times, like the sex after the big fight. How many times have we heard from our patients and friends how they have to reject a possible mate because they seem to be normal, they seem to just want to love and be loved. They would not know what to do if they did not choose the complicated, hurtful, erotic, intense shame of intimacy and lust. We in the groups spend an enormous amount of time trying to talk, listen, and see the shame in our lives and in our souls.

What keeps Sharon hidden in the shadows in the group? Why is she acting like she doesn't belong? What keeps Debra having one foot in and one foot out? What keeps Marlene, always charged, always erotic, always daring new adventures? What keeps Owen, the wise one of the group, terrified to join us as a happy kid having fun in my fantasy lap? What keeps Jim from staying in the group and competing with me for the women in the group? Why is he always the student, never the teacher? Why does Leah keep denying that she wants to have a man like me, yet feels tied up and shamed by these feelings?

How can Barney, a long-term patient in many different groups of mine over time, make peace with his powerful loving feelings, and yet does not feel that I truly understand his regression when his sons unravel. Why can't I make it better? Why can't Sharon just accept her partner's childlike behavior and call it a day? Why do I keep harping on how she is living with this situation? Why don't I just fly away? "You should be grieving instead of tormenting all of us with these questions," she says. I keep reiterating that they are trying to call their Passionate Bad Fit a good one. Their regressions would not let them. We all went back to the earliest time of life, before words, just body-to-body and insides-to-insides. What do you think my inside is like now, and has it changed?

The groups were basically in the same place with each other. Their work together for many years built a comradery and trust and openness in the group. They were stable and began to enjoy their newfound identity in a family. They never had a stable, healthy identity in their families. They never had family disagreements without chaos. Their experience was captured beautifully when I would ask them to describe their family dinners or Sunday lunches. They were able to finally laugh at the absurdity of those events, and how small they felt to themselves and to the family members.

There were two new members in two of the three groups, and both left prematurely, after 6–9 months. They both left as we got into how they have carried the worst part of their parents in their life and called it love and closeness. I may have been too caught up in the power of our work together and did not spend enough time with the newer members. I may have erred by not trying to relive the earliest wordless years with them and me. Maybe I was too tired, exhausted by my grief and needing to keep being excellent with my groups. I may have put myself in a Passionate Bad fit that did not protect me did not slow me down and just enjoy being held in their laps. In my own way, I rejected their comfort and instead landed in my own powerful Passionate Bad Fit.

It was looking at their early mergers and how it led them to live in Passionate Bad Fits. The losses were hard for the groups and they questioned my theories and how I care for them. They asked, "Why would anyone leave this place? What could we have done better to keep them? What could you have done to keep them? You got manipulated by one of the members who left. How did this happen?"

"There are better con men out there than I am." I admit I got taken in by him, and I asked the same questions. But I will not carry his shame about leaving as he had left his mother years before and never spoke with her until she died. That was his Omnipotent Child, and we became his mother, and he had to leave her and that part of him that was his unfaithful mother. He also wanted us to feel his shame and degradation, when she mistreated him, when she sexualized the relationship, and when he felt she had betrayed him. He was good at projective identification, because the group all felt that. One woman in particular felt betrayed by him, because she let herself have intense vivid sexual fantasies of him. How could she not? He was a pro, and she was a neophyte in his world. He, interestingly though, did not really want to hear how attracted she was toward him. He filled the time with his minute-to-minute conquests over women, and then his rejecting them. The group was both his mother and the little boy, which the group carried for him.

I tended to make a big deal of what the little kids in the group had to carry with what was inside their parents or the family. How painful it was to be the chosen one, the adored one, and, most importantly, the grandiose one. It was very hard for the groups to hear how magnificent their burden was, and then how magnificent their Passionate Bad Fit was to them.

I had a group member who gloriously told the group how he had built a real monument to his hamsters as he watched them enjoy the thrill of riding in the monument he built. He described it in detail and was shocked that he had let his animals play out his own monument to his being left out, to his never being able to find the right woman for himself, and for his awkward social communication skills. He always got members to be angry, sorry, guilty, and shameful about not being able to love him the way he wanted. He did best when he played a fantasy child-hood game with one of the women in the group. But he could not do it again the next time we met. The little boy in him was too close to the moments of grandiosity and rupture that he kept reliving in his adult life.

I learned how the need to recapture the lost grandiosity of infanthood for both parent and child was unconscious and played a great role in maintaining the stability of the Passionate Bad Fit identity. The grandiosity needs to both run the show and demand a separate identity and wishes and yet needs the merger with the elusive other grandiosity. This was hard work for all of us, and each group did it in their own special way. One group played it out with each other.

Lonny keeps choosing to live with his wife, who has made it clear to him and the group that he comes in third, with her older child first. This keeps his "rejection button" alive and always operating. He is carrying the shame of his mother and father, who were trying to be parents when that was not what they really wanted. The thought of taking a risk and trying a separation from his wife is immediately transformed into his rejection button. "No one will like me, I'm afraid to be alone," and with prompting from me and group, "I am most afraid of giving up my rejection button, to find a different partner who really loves me and whom I can really love. I am getting older, aren't I?" He is only now becoming aware of how he is the frustrating, rejecting mother and father to the group, as his little boy was in his real life. He is beginning to realize how he lives in the group, holding on to the wonderful isolating grandiosity of rejection. He is still in shock about this idea of himself in the group. It is all there in the group, we just have to see it and use it properly to inform, educate, and change their behavior.

The group's dilemma, as we get closer to shifting to a Passionate Good Fit, is taking a risk either in or outside the group, or in their ability to bring in dreams, allow fantasies about each other, etc. They have to take a risk to notice what happens to their encrusted identity, which is absolutely imperative for their growth in the group. Without genuine risk-taking, I do not believe that the members will really be able to live in the Passionate Good Fit and hold it and claim it as their new identity. They would have to give up and develop a new relationship with their Omnipotent Child and the way it manages conflict, love, hate, identity, the body, etc.

This experience of risk-taking leaves patients without a stable identity that has been the centerpiece and its grandiosity all rolled up in one. They feel homeless, helpless, terrified, angry, taken in, and manipulated, and it is like being in a valley where you really cannot see other sides. The group is the best place I know to be the holder of this exquisite agony and loss of identity. I know how to be the holder of this exquisite agony and loss of identity. I too have let myself feel the Omnipotent Child in me. When I write this book, a part of me feels disloyal to the work that Sheila and I did for this book. I attune to her loneliness underground sometimes, when I feel lost, unregulated, and angry at the world. The groups contain me, nurture me, and allow me to continue to grow through this difficult experience.

The group learns to hold, have empathy, laugh at the comic scenes as this despair is presented and recounted. The mighty have fallen, the vulnerable shrug and say, "What's the big deal? I've lived in this valley all my life. Just get used to it." Now they start asking each other, "How would you define your Passionate Bad Fit?" They do not want to be alone in the valley. They reach out to each other in a very different way, like the early wordless experience in their life. Only they have put words to it. "We need to be inside each other." They feel much closer to each other and talk about group solidarity, group unity, and the group family. They start to wonder whether I will continue working. "You are much older now, and have recently lost your wife. Can you take good care of yourself?" The unhealthy narcissism begins to shift to a healthier narcissism, without shame. They start communicating with each other through their insides. They begin to tell each other what is inside of them.

> Marlene confesses to feeling that her mother wanted to eat and swallow her up, and how she has had relationships in which she ate and then discarded the man. Debra says she cannot remember dreams, because she does not trust herself. She has been asexual because she has sadomasochistic fantasies that have paralyzed her sexuality.
>
> Barney is able to acknowledge how attracted he was to the sister–mother fights in his youth. He let the group know what a bully he can be in his business. He felt free enough in the group to reenact his experience with me about how he feels when one of his children terrifies, enrages, and humiliates him. He feels that he cannot do anything right with his son, and this has been going on forever. He will periodically start a session with how much he cares about me and how angry and disappointed he is with me. How much I have helped him over the years, but "I have to admit that you cannot get it right, you confuse me and your comments make me feel small, judged and humiliated. I don't know

why you do that to me. I'm your longest patient, and you know how much I need you, yet your answers to how to help me with my adult child seem intellectual and don't take into context my reactions to his threats. He, my child, keeps threatens suicide, and all you can say is that he is very unstable, he has an unstable identity, and he needs to be hospitalized or at least in a long-term treatment situation. Your comments, especially those that point out how regressed I get when he threatens me, only leave me cold and helpless to help my child. You have said that I act as if we are merged and you are both the threatening and regressed father and adult child." I say, "You have merged with him, and when he regresses, so do you." "The issue is not what terrible harmful things did I do with this child of mine, but why and how did I get so merged with him?" "I have been trying to help you see the merger, which explains the degree of regression you feel when he terrifies and shames you. You didn't want to be like your father, too self-involved, and you saw how your sister and mother shared a special closeness through their fights. You didn't know how to raise a child, how close is close, how do you love without being depleted and not getting what you personally need. I can understand your fury with me." "What kind of answer is that?" "I don't have an easy recipe for cure, only questions that I ask and try to answer." "You always make me feel terrible. I cannot sleep at night, I want to hate you, I feel that you have cheated me."

Over the last two or three years, he has lived in this re-creation. The group helped him when they said that he sounded like his child and, "You want Stewart to know how your child makes you feel. You are him and Stewart is you." I, in fact, became more aware of how painful it has been for him, as it is for me to see him claw at me and let me know how I failed him and hurt him, and clearly, painfully, see my intellectual comments did not touch him the way I thought they would. I let him know that and will pay more attention to how I can get us on the same page about his terrible experience with his adult child.

Patients went around the room to see how they have projected themselves into the other group members. Projective identification is one of the tools that I and the group use all the time, and try to get the re-creations that I just talked about to happen as much as possible. In my theory, these experiences are also a way to try to give back the carried shame to the parent. When this is examined in that way, the experience of the projective identification takes on new meaning for the group in their advancement of trying to move from the Passionate Bad Fit to the Passionate Good Fit. The reduction in shame is crucial to allow this transformation to grow and become a part of their risk-taking,

I strongly support this adventure, because naming it gives it a reality that helps make it conscious. I remembered how I could never define my father other than as a powerful, scary man who could not be talked to and terrified me. I did not share this with my groups. But he was unnamed until I saw a great movie with William Bendix, who looked like my father to me, sweaty, hairy, strong arms, and silent. I suddenly knew who my father was: The Hairy Ape. I was so relieved. Naming helps by informing us how to relate to this newly named person. You have a better chance to know the insides of that person, and, in particular, his shame, successes, and motivation, and how he tries to love and command at the same time. You can take things from him without shame and have the pleasure of picking and choosing over time. When I was younger, I used to go into their bedroom, fish around in his pants pockets on the chair, and steal money from him. I learned how to have a really hot soup that burned my palate, how to keep working, how to be responsible, how to be the leader, how to not keep myself alone (even though I have a tendency to stay on the sidelines until asked in).

The groups needed to name their Omnipotent Child to each other and live with the consequences. This was the big risk-taking in the groups, as well as reaching out beyond themselves to attach to others. To try to create a new family in the group requires an acknowledgment of how your bad fit prevents you from joining in, and allows you to replicate the loneliness, helplessness, and the masochism and sadism in the family to exist, and define the family. The group is always looking to see how some members will choose the Passionate Bad Fit over the risk of a different family, with a different leader—me. I make that abundantly clear to the group from its inception, that I am the most important person in the group, even though my role may change.

Stan, a married man in his eighties, comes to treatment because he is not happy, and he thinks his wife does not like him anymore. He cannot tell you why that would be the case, because he can't remember his early childhood anymore. I had worked with him and his wife many years ago, and was struck by her masochistic surrender to him and his unhealthy narcissism. He carried with him the narcissism of his rejecting and critical mother, and his father's letting him take care of his mother, while the father fished and became a very respected professional. Steve has become filled with his parents' shame, and his own shame about his children. His strength was his practice, but he has retired and, along with some physical issues, has hit a very low point in his self-esteem. He tries never to notice his internal life, and in the group tends to tell us stories, never answers direct questions, and clearly is distressed. Lynn, out of her newfound healthy narcissism, says that I am not helping him attach to us in the group, and my asking him about his past and present life is missing the point. "Well taken," I say. Lynn then tries to get him to notice and listen to what she is saying to him, and keeps bringing him back to the group and his attachments. As with her parents and life journey, she gives up easily and tries to find a newer exciting fantasy object to keep her in denial about how her parents did not give her what she needed in the large family she was raised in. She tried to be powerful and win medals, but failed again to capture her mother's attention. She has equated success with that failure, and therefore will not try to reach for healthy successes. We uncovered a part of her Omnipotent Child, and I hope that in the remaining time I have left in the group to appreciate that she has captured me and others the group, and can that be enough? Can that success ever shine as bright as the failure to capture the elusive mother? At times, she becomes the elusive mother in the room, by not being dependable, coming late, and saying that she has had to put up with me and the group for many years.

Part Two

How did I decide to let my groups know that I was going to give up my groups, six in all, at the end of December 2022? In the two years since my wife died, I have learned how to be alone, how to take good care of myself, and have begun to make friends at my living complex. I started to think of women in my life and started to date someone. I was struck by how there was a big difference between how she saw and felt me and how I felt about her. At the end of the first year here, I developed some medical issues that led to surgery and repeated visits to the hospital. I was extremely weakened by this and felt humiliated by this mess in my body. I continued to run the groups, but let them know that I was not feeling well, and that I was tired, did not have the stamina I was used to, and would continue to work as long as I did not become a burden to them. We worked like that for a while, and then I began to notice that I at times forgot some evening groups until the last moment. It was clear that I was being told something by my mind and body, and I needed to listen. I was quite honest with my training groups and, because we met only twice a year, I did not have to confront my state of the union. But my administrative skills, which were never very good, really deteriorated and led to confusion among the group members and for me. I journeyed into self-pity a lot and then would shake it off, like an annoying bug. But still I did not pay enough attention to my condition. I eventually recovered from my infectious body and began to feel like my old self. My children insisted that I get daily help, which I reluctantly did, and my spirits rose. I talk often with my colleagues about this, and they all say that retirement soon makes a great deal of sense. "You deserve it. You worked all your life. You will still be Dr. Group to us."

   In one of my Tuesday night groups, I made an error with a patient and was called on it by her and the group. I was humiliated, shamed, and scared. The dreaded side of my own Passionate Bad Fit was arriving, and how could I stop it from taking over, as it had earlier in my life? The group asked how I was feeling, and said that they were concerned about my eyes closing on occasion in the group, and my not remembering a story that was told the previous session, and that they thought that I looked too thin.

   Along with their concerns, the groups felt that, even as I got older, I seemed to have more wisdom in my comments, in my theory, and in putting what we talk about in the context of our work together, which is finally making a great deal of sense to us.

   We are not living in a Passionate Bad fit with you now, but want to make sure we do not end up there. We want to applaud our newfound healthy narcissism, our taking risks that we never thought we could, and our love and tenderness for you and how you stood the test of time, and taught us how we can deal with the test of time. You taught us about the shame we carried, and how different life is inside of us without shame.

The love, the adulation I felt, was magnificent. But I always knew there was another side to it that was not being talked about. I tried to help them talk of their disappointment with me, their anger at the parent that they could not rely on, the feeling that they may have to rescue me from myself and my destiny. As the group continued, it became crystal clear to me that it was time to retire. I thought about it as the group was talking to me and others and, to my amazement, I announced to the group, in that session, that I would be giving up the groups in one year. I did not expect that to happen. The groups had become the family I lost when my wife died. How could I do this during a group session? Was it a Bad Fit or a Good Fit? Was I most real with my groups, more than with others? Have I not grieved enough for Sheila? Have I given into a theatrical part of myself? I always wanted to be an actor or a baseball announcer saying "Going, going, gone" when someone hits a home run. Did I need their adoration to carry me through my retirement? Did trying to write a book about my work finally let me feel that I had a hobby to play with during retirement? Did I really like myself better, as I too had a great deal of the shame that I was carrying from my parents and my failures?

These questions helped me redefine myself and take a hard look at who I am now and who I was earlier in my life. Do I really want to live with someone now, or do I need my freedom, which I never let myself notice before? How powerful am I? How passive and accommodating can I slip into being? As the groups were trying to live in the Passionate Good Fit and deal with their constant undoing of this Fit, I too could empathize with them, as I would go back and forth about what fit I will live in. Unconsciously, the groups and I were living inside each other. We were developing a new language to counter the wordless earliest life experiences. There are therapists who think that, over time, groups will take care of this earliest period. I disagree. I think you need to start with it, and structure your work around the earliest misattunements and the power of shame to keep the Passionate Bad Fit alive.

The groups and I are becoming a form of merged identities, trying to help each other to live in the Passionate Good Fit and point out the Omnipotent Child in all of us. In this context, the groups become more acquainted with their undoing of the move "to the other side of the river." I have been struck by my use of biblical terms as I help the group describe and name their behavior. I guess working on this level felt biblical to me—ancient, wise, and present.

How did the group react to the announcement that in one year I will be stopping as the therapist? There was a surprise, followed by an awareness that it was going to happen sooner or later. They were pleased with the long notice but also felt that they could not take it seriously enough because of the long notice. They felt they needed to try harder, work faster, and really get better. For whom? Me or you? No one dropped out at that time. I also said that I would not be taking on any new patients now. "We are who we are together," I said. I told them that I would let them know about my medical life, if it comes up in my work. Over time, they were able to talk sheepishly of how upset they would be when my eyes would close, or when I forgot a session and had to be reminded by phone of it. They wanted to know if they could see other members outside the group when they left. I said, "No, it doesn't work." They wanted to know what will happen to the group after I leave. I told them that they could choose to stay together, and I would find therapists who could take my place. They also could go their separate ways and I would refer them to other therapists for group or individual therapy. There were many questions and answers during this period of time.

There was one member who left, after I had agreed to see her former husband in one of my groups. I had worked with both of them as a couple and then each had come into one of my groups separately. She was furious that I did not consult her about this decision I made, and she could not bear his being in treatment with me and trying to control her life. Up to the point they had separated, she had continued with the group and with an occasional individual session. The major issue, as she stated it, was how she cannot seem to settle with another man in her life, even though she had dated and been somewhat serious with some men. I wondered whether her romantic feelings toward me had interfered with her search for a man. She tended to agree, but would not go further with it unless I would bring it up. The rest of her divorced life had gone well, dealing with her two kids, and money issues with her ex-husband. She tended to be not as attached to the other members of the group, and tended to at times be a little girl twirling her hair. She liked to bring in stories that did not have any real openings for others to react to. She was there, but not there. She was able to acknowledge that it was her way to let the group know how she felt in her house. She was there as an appendage to her mother, and a negotiable item to her father. Her only real life as a kid was in summer camp. She repeatedly wanted permission to leave the group, which I thought was her feeling as if she was imprisoned with us, as well as with her husband, and is still searching for that summer camp of freedom, independence, and grandiosity without selling her soul to her parents to get it. This was her Omnipotent Child in all its glory. She would bring in very rich and elegant fantasies of her life, at which the group marveled at first, and then were able to see the grandiosity that concealed the little girl's terrifying capture and imprisonment. She did finally deal forcefully with her mother and father and got more separation from them, but she still could not find the right man.

About four months into the last year, I made the mistake of taking her ex-husband into one of my groups. She stormed and acted like a jealous spouse that I had cheated on. She gave two weeks' notice, and this time was adamant that she could no longer work with me if I treated her ex-husband. Why did I bring him in? Did I want her to leave the group? Was I getting more uncomfortable talking with her, and interpreting some of her behaviors in the group as a deep powerful attraction and fantasy life with me? She would at times agree, and wanted to know why she could not find me out there.

The dilemma of being the object of desire is a powerful issue that again does not get enough attention at meetings and in the literature. Being the object of desire is crucial to both my technique and my theory of group psychotherapy.

Chapter 21

Retirement and Ending the Groups

Stewart and Lee Talk

This conversation took place on 1/28/23, after Stewart had shut down all 6 of his groups: the 3 training groups and 3 regular weekly therapy groups.

LK: Have you finished the process of shutting down?

SA: Yes, everything is closed. It was quite an experience.

LK: Let's dive into that.

SA: The regular weekly groups, not the training groups, each had about 6 or 8 members. We met once a week for an hour and a half. I gave them all one year's notice, to say that I was retiring.

LK: Was there reaction from the members when you gave them one year's notice?

SA: Absolutely. A lot of them said, "Well, we can understand, Stewart, because there are time when your eyes close during the group." I said, "Yes, that's one of the reasons." "And there are times when you have forgotten the group, and we had to call to get you there." I said,

> Yes, I remember that. I put this all together, and I realized that as I've aged the most difficult thing for me to gin up is my stamina. I don't think I fully realized what it was like for me to run all these groups for an hour and a half every week, and keep all of you more than just in my mind, but inside of me.

LK: It sounds like they were expecting it.

SA: They were, and they weren't. What they said was,

> We don't really care if your eyes close, we don't really care if you forget a meeting if we can get and you'll come to the meeting. We think that, even under these circumstances, you are the best, and we don't want to give you up. What we've noticed is, even if your eyes close, you don't forget a goddamn thing. You remember everything about us.

I said,

> What I used to remember about you, all the people in your life: uncles, aunts, parents, siblings, spouses, children. I don't remember them now at all. What I remember now is who you are in the transferences in this

DOI: 10.4324/9781032705835-26

group. And my lack of stamina has never affected that. There are times when I feel tired, and I don't want to come to the group. I'm somewhere chatting with people and I forget. Then it's 5 o'clock, and oh my God, I've got the group.

I was trying to be as honest as I could to all three of these groups as to why I made this decision, and I also said that the decision occurred in one of the groups I was running. I had made some comments to one of the members of the group that I really should not have made. It showed lack of discipline, it showed sloppiness on my part, it showed irreverence, and it was just not right, and the group really jumped on me for that, and they had a perfect right to, but it made me think, while in the group, that session, that I shouldn't be doing this anymore.

> I do not want you all to end up having to take care of me. I will not have that! And I know that all of you, deep inside, would love to be able to be my lap, to take care of me. I will not have that. That's not what you're here for. You're here to take care of yourselves.

We would talk a lot about that, and there was a lot of anger, at some point, and some people would say, "Look. Let's cut the shit. You don't love us enough to stay. If you really loved us, like you keep saying you do, you'd stay, but you're walking away, like a traitor." And I said,

> Well, we at times have to be disloyal in order to grow, and I am being disloyal. I'm aware of that. But I have to look after myself, too, and become a model for how you look after yourself. I have no interest in being dragged out of here as a grade-D therapist. I am a grade-A therapist, a great therapist, and that's how I want to be remembered.

We kept talking about my decision, they would not drop it. It came down to, "If you really love me, you would not leave me," plain and simple.

I would remind them periodically, like at six months, that I would be retiring in another six months. "Now what we have to decide is, what do you do next? Where do you all go? Does the group survive without me?" I said that what I wanted to do was, if the groups were interested, to continue the groups without me, with a new therapist. I contacted three therapists here in town, who I know from my training groups, they all know my theory, they all know my style, it's two men and a woman, and we worked out the time. They all wanted to hold on to their regular time, as part of their identity. When I gave the therapists the day and time, two of them dropped out, because they couldn't do it. So one man is taking over two of the groups, and one is disbanding.

They asked me what it would be like for me, and I said that I would be ending all my groups, and on one hand it's very exciting to me, but I have to figure out on the other hand, what is so exciting about ending everything?

Why aren't you just sad? I said, "I'm very sad about not being part of you, and you being part of me, but I'm also very happy and relieved about ending the responsibility."

LK: It must feel like a new kind of freedom.

SA: Yes. I told them, "I will have to get used to it, just like all of you. It's a change in my identity, and who will I be without these groups?" I've decided to be available for another year to see some people from the group individually if they want to. There was a lot of fuss about that, which was, "Well, that's not really an ending."

There was one patient, a woman whose mother had been very engulfing.

She wanted to swallow me, and make me disappear, and that's a death, isn't it? I want an ending with you, where I don't disappear, you don't disappear, we are both able to stand up and say goodbye. I want a clear ending.

There were a lot of dreams of loss. Some typical dreams form the groups: I lost my car, I couldn't find my purse, I lost my wallet. But then I said, "But what about the other side? There might be some relief. I'm a tough son-of-a-bitch. I make a lot of demands on all of you. I'm not easy. I make you work." Many times, people have said I've been too harsh, or too rough. I think they were right, and I've apologized.

I take this work very seriously. When I see someone futzing around, and not taking the next step, and the next risk, that really gets me going, and I want to know why. What's the risk going to be for them when I leave? The risk is going to be, can they survive? Can they make it work with a new therapist? I've tried to accentuate all the healthy changes that people have made while in the group.

There are risks to develop a new identity, and risks to be disloyal to me, and the biggest risk of all is, can you cross over the river and start living the Passionate Good Fit? The big risk is disloyalty to the old bad fit.

LK: I want to hear more about you and your experience ending your practice.

SA: It was not easy to find therapists to take over the groups. I was shocked that two of them said, "I can't do it. I can't do those times." One therapist took two groups. The third group decided that they did not want to work with a new therapist, partly because they thought that the group had done its job. I agreed with them about that.

During that time, a lot was happening to me, because I was letting myself meet someone. I met a woman here, and she had a wonderful smile, and something developed. That was a big deal for me, because I was shifting identities from being alone, or being in a difficult relationship, to being with someone who was easy. I realized that I like easy. So while the groups are ending, I'm starting a whole new relationship, with a woman who is different from any woman I've ever been involved with. My theory has invaded me as much as it has my patients, and I have been disloyal to my own past.

LK: It seems to me that you don't have to work with your groups, and you don't have to work with your partner either.

SA: Every now and then I would say to myself, "You sure you know what you're doing, Stewart? This woman isn't driving you crazy. Can you live with that?"

LK: There must be something wrong with it!

SA: There's no question that it's related to ending the groups and developing a new identity, and taking a big risk. Everyone in the groups has been taking big risks in this year of ending.

LK: The first risk is joining the group in the first place. Anyone who joins a group is taking a big risk.

SA: Yes. So they've taken risks, and made big changes, and the question is, can they hold on to the progress? They've spent a lot of time in the last six months undoing, and when you cross over into the good fit, you have a new identity, you can feel lost, and not sure who you are. People have dreams of being stuck in a valley between two mountains, and they couldn't get up on top.

LK: So they're tempted to go back.

SA: Yes. I call it "the siren song." In this last six months period, one patient said, "I know what you're doing. You're making sure that our toolbox is full, and also that we begin to understand why we go back." I said, "Yes, and what you need now is a radar, that starts beeping to let you know that you're hearing the siren song. Different people have different radars. It's already in your body." One guy said he would stop breathing, and I said, "That's your radar." So I turned the theory into something mechanical, in a way, something logistical, something mechanical. And then we talk about that struggle, not to cross back over into the old bad fit.

LK: Was it different with the training groups?

SA: I think they were more defended. The therapy groups met every week, The training groups met every six months. A very different experience. In the therapy groups, they didn't know each other outside of group. in the training groups, they all knew each other. There, the focus was on what they were going to do in the six months between meetings. Those groups met for 25 or 30 years, so we had a lot of sessions, but also a lot of time between sessions.

LK: How were those groups different for you?

SA: it's been hard for me to define it. I think I felt more relief in ending them, because they became problematic when we switched to Zoom during the pandemic. Administratively, it was a real pain in the ass. I recruited someone from the group to be my secretary, my administrator, to get them together. I admitted that I couldn't deal with it.

I think there was not as much progress in the training groups, although some people did a wonderful job of changing their lives around. But it was always cluttered with a lot of noise. They were stuck with six months of trying to figure out what was going on in themselves, because a lot would happen in the weekend meeting.

LK: What was the rationale for so much time between meetings?

SA: At the time, no one was doing training groups, so I had to construct it myself. Someone asked for a training group, and I asked her when she could meet, and she said that people would be coming in from all over, and it would be expensive, so maybe twice a year. Sometimes we would discuss going to three times a year, but it never got taken up. Maybe that was because of me, because I didn't want to meet three times a year. It was awesome to work in the groups, but not easy to get them together. At the end of each session, we would try to come up with a date for the next time, and it was always filled with a lot of anger. "You never pick my date, you always [ick someone else's date." Who's your favorite? Who do you love?

      They tried not to have too much interaction between them in the six-month breaks, but sometimes they would see each other, and there was always the hint that someone was having sex with someone else. I had to be a detective, I had to smell it out.

LK: Did that actually happen?

SA: I don't think so. I think they got high together, but I don't think anything sexual happened.

      In the undoing, they go back to a toxic merger, to the origins of the Passionate Bad Fit, and the major ingredient that drives it is shame. What most people have said, in both the weekly therapy groups and the training groups, is how different their lives are without shame driving them. One thing I'm most proud of, that made the biggest difference in their lives, is that they moved from unhealthy narcissism, which is fueled by shame, and the Passionate Bad Fit, to healthy narcissism, which is *not* fueled by shame. It's fueled by energy, by success, accomplishment, creativity, by healthy stuff. At the same time, there was also a tremendous change in how they experienced their bodies. In the Passionate Bad Fit, the body contains all the shame and the negative impulses, and they end up with their body being an enemy, not an ally. As they begin to reduce the shame in their lives, they notice that they feel better about their body. Both the women and the men talk about it.

      I spent a lot of time with all these groups talking about, where is shame in your life? And where is shame in the group? And how do we deal with it? I never stopped talking about shame. Whenever I smelled it, felt, or sensed it, I brought it up.

LK: In these last few months of the groups, you're trying to remind them of all the things they worked on in the prior years.

SA: It's a way to show them that they now have a toolbox that's filled with the proper tools. They have a radar system that alerts them. They have a healthy narcissism, and a healthy grandiosity, and therefore they can appreciate *my* grandiosity, and take some from me, because I have plenty to give.

      At the very end, with the local groups, I invited them into my apartment, to meet for the last time. That was quite an experience! I was wondering, how am I going to take what's inside them for me? Just as I ask them how they're going to take what's inside of me that's good for them. I decided unconsciously that the best way to show them that I was taking them inside was to invite them into my home. It was fantastic. There are pictures of me as a kid. With people I worked with, when they ended treatment, and left the group, they usually gave me a glass figurine. I had them spread out all over the apartment. They said, "This reminds me of your office." I said, "Yes, it's very similar."

LK: You're breaking the cardinal rules.

SA: Yes, I am. I struggled with the decision. Do I have enough room? What does it mean? Then I got rid of "what does it mean." It'll mean whatever it means. We're at the point that it's a risk that *I'm* taking. I'm going to show them that I can take a risk. But I wondered, where does it fit in my theory? I didn't do it with the training groups.

LK: I'm remembering that some of the people I interviewed from the training groups told me that when you first started developing your theory you would talk about taking people into your body.

SA: That's right. It's a good example of it. I ended up going back to my original work, in a way.

LK: You came full circle.

SA: I did. I came full circle.

References

Agazarian, Y. M. (1997). *System centered therapy*. New York: Guilford Press.

Aledort, S. L. (1994). A model for the development of an analytic culture in intensive multi-weekly group psychoanalysis. Presented at National Group Psychotherapy Institute Conference Washington, DC.

Aledort, S. L. (2002). The omnipotent child syndrome: The role of the passionately held bad fits in the formation of identity. *International Journal of Group Psychotherapy, 52*, 67–88.

Aledort, S. L. (2003). Fleshing out the omnipotent child in group psychotherapy. *Group, 27*, 151–167.

Aledort, S. L. (2008). A model for the development of an analytic culture in intensive multi-weekly group psychoanalysis. In *Windows into today's group therapy* (pp. 177–189). National Group Psychotherapy Institute of the Washington School of Psychiatry. East Sussex: Routledge/Taylor & Francis.

Aledort, S. L. (2009). Excitement: A crucial marker for group psychotherapy. *Group, 33*, 45–63.

Alonso, A., & Rutan, J. S. (1988). The experience of shame and the restoration of self-respect in group therapy. *International Journal of Group Psychotherapy, 38*, 3–14.

Alonso, A., & Rutan, S. (1993). Character change in group therapy. *International Journal of Group Psychotherapy, 43*, 439–451.

Bateman, A., & Fonagy, P. (2013). Mentalization-based treatment. *Psychoanalytic Inquiry, 33*(6), 595–613.

Beebe, B. (2000). Co-constructing the mother-infant distress. The microsynchrony of maternal impingement and infant avoidance in the face-to-face encounter. *Psychoanalytic Inquiry, 20*, 412–440.

Beebe, B., & Lachman, F. M. (2002). *Infant research and adult treatment: Co-creating interactions*. Hillsdale, NJ: Analytic Press.

Beebe, B., Lachman, F., & Jaffe, J. (1997). Mother-infant interaction structures and presymbolic self- and object representations. *Psychoanalytic Dialogues, 7*, 133–182.

Boston Change Process Study Group (1998). Report I. Non-interpretive mechanisms in psychoanalytic therapy. The something more than interpretation. *International Journal of Psychoanalysis, 79*, 908–919.

Brynolf Lyon, K., Berley, R., & Klassen, K. (2012). Unbearable states of mind in group psychotherapy: Disassociation, Mentalization and the clinician's stance. *Group, 36*(4), 267–282.

Chuah, T. (1986). Developmental imagery: An antidote to annihilation in the countertransference. In *Current issues in psychoanalytic practice* (Ed. H. Strean) (pp. 75–93). New York: Haworth Press.

Cohen, B. (2000). Intersubjectivity and narcissism in group psychotherapy: How feedback works. *International Journal of Group Psychotherapy, 50*, 163–181.

Cohen, E. S., & Rogovin, S. A., with Thompson, A. (2000). *Couple fits*. New York: Berkley Publishing Group.

Durkin, H. E., & Glatzer, H. T. (1997). Transference neurosis in group psychotherapy: The concept and the reality. *International Journal of Group Psychotherapy, 47*, 183–199.

Erikson, E. (1969). *Gandhi's truth: On the origins of militant nonviolence*. New York: Norton.

Fonagy, P. (1999). Points of contact and divergence between psychoanalytic and attachment theories: Is psychoanalytic theory truly different? *Psychoanalytic Inquiry, 19*, 448–441.

Frankl, V. E. (1984). *Man's search for meaning*. New York & London: Simon & Schuster.

Frederickson, J. (2000). There's something "youey" about you. The polyphonic unity of personhood. *Contemporary Psychoanalysis, 36*, 587–617.

Freedman, D. (1989). Maturational and developmental issues in the first year. In S. Greenspan & G. Pollock (Ed.), *The course of life, Vol. 1: Infancy* (pp. 293–320). Madison, CT: International Universities Press.

Gans, J. (2018). *Difficult topics in group psychotherapy: My journey from shame to courage*. New York: Routledge.

Gans, J., & Alonso, A. (1998). Difficult patients: Their construction in group therapy. *International Journal of Group Psychotherapy, 48*, 311–327.

Hendrick, I. (1943). Work and the pleasure principle. *Psychoanalytic Quarterly, 12*, 311–329.

Kandel, E. (1998). A new intellectual framework for psychiatry. *American Journal of Psychiatry, 155*, 457–469.

Kauff, P. (1997). Transference and regression in and beyond analytic group psychotherapy: Revisiting some timeless thoughts. *International Journal of Group Psychotherapy, 47*, 201–210.

Kernberg, O. F. (2001). Object relations, affects, and drives: Toward a new synthesis. *Psychoanalytic Inquiry, 21*, 604–620.

Klein, M. (1946). Notes on some schizoid mechanisms. In Ernest Jones (Ed.) *Developments in psychoanalysis* (pp. 292–320). London: Hogarth Press.

Kohut, H. (1978). Thoughts on narcissism and narcissistic rage. In P. H. Ornstein (Ed.) *The search for the self: Selected writings of Heinz Kohut: 1950-1978* (Vol. 2). Madison, CT: International Universities Press.

Kohut, H. (1984). *How does analysis cure?* (Ed. A. Goldberg & P. Stepansky). Chicago, IL: University of Chicago Press.

Leszcz, M. (1989). Group psychotherapy of the characterologically difficult patient. *International Journal of Group Psychotherapy, 39*, 311–335.

Lichtenberg, J. (1999). Discussion. *Psychoanalytic Inquiry, 19*, 647–662.

Livingston, M. S. (2003). Vulnerability, affect and depth in group psychotherapy. *Group, 23*, 646–677.

Livingston, M. S. (2004). *Vulnerable moments: Deepening the therapeutic process*. Northvale, NJ: Jason Aronson.

Livingston, L. R. P. (2006). No place to hide: The group leader's moments of shame. *International Journal of Group Psychotherapy, 56*(3), 307–324.

Mahler, M. S. (1968). *On human symbiosis and the vicissitudes of individuation*. New York: International Universities Press.

Mahler, M. S., Pine, F., & Bergman, A. (1975). *The psychological birth of the human infant*. New York: Basic Books.

Malcolm, J. (1981). *Psychoanalysis: The impossible profession*. New York: Knopf.

Mazer, H., & Rako, S. (1980). *Semrad: The heart of a therapist*. Northvale, NJ: Jason Aronson.

Mitchell, S. A. (1993). *Hope and dread in psychoanalysis*. New York: Basic Books.

Mollon, P. (2003). *Shame and jealousy*: London: Karnac.

Morrison, A. P. (1989). *Shame: The underside of narcissism*. New York: Routledge/Taylor & Francis Group.

Motherwell, L. (Ed.) (2014). *Complex dilemmas in group therapy: Pathways to resolution*, 2nd ed.). London and New York: Routledge.

Nitsun, M. (1996). *The anti-group*. London: Routledge.

Nitsun, M. (2006). *The group as an object of desire: Exploring sexuality in group therapy*. London and New York: Routledge.

Ormont, L. R. (1992). *The group experience from theory to practice*. New York: St. Martin's Press.

Ormont, L. R. (2006). Keeping the group flourishing. *Group, 30*(3), 205–216.

Phillips, A. (1993). *On kissing, tickling and being bored. Psychoanalytic essays on the unexamined life*. Cambridge, MA: Harvard University Press.

Pine, F. (1985). *Developmental theory and clinical process*. New Haven, CT: Yale University Press.

Pine, F. (1994). The era of separation–individuation. *Psychoanalytic Inquiry, 14*, 4–25.

Rako, S., & Mazer, H. (1983). *Semrad: The heart of a therapist*. Northvale, NJ and London: Jason Aronson.

Rice, C. A., Shapiro, E. L., & Shay, J. J. (2011). The death of a group therapist and the survival of the group. *International Journal of Group Psychotherapy, 61*(2), 176–195.

Roller, B., & Nelson, V. (1999). Group psychotherapy treatment of borderline personalities. *International Journal of Group Psychotherapy, 49*, 369–386.

Rosenthal, L. (2006). The re-enactment of familial roles as resistance in group psychotherapy. *Group, 30*(3), 185–204.

Rutan, J. S., Stone, W. S., & Shay, J. J. (2007). *Psychodynamic group psychotherapy*, 4th ed. New York & London: Guilford Press.

Sacks, O. (1983). *Awakenings*. New York: Dutton.

Sacks, O. (1993). *A leg to stand on*. New York: Touchstone.

Sacks, O. (2007). *Musicophilia*. New York & London: Knopf.

Scharff, J. (2001). Case presentation: The object relations approach. *Psychoanalytic Inquiry, 21*, 469–483.

Schermer, V. (2000). Contributions of object relations theory and self psychology to relational psychology and group psychotherapy. *International Journal of Group Psychotherapy, 50*, 199–217.

Schlachet, P. (1998). Discussion of "Difficult Patients." *International Journal of Group Psychotherapy, 48*, 327–333.

Schore, A. (2002a). Dysregulation of the right brain: A fundamental mechanism of traumatic attachment and the psychopathogenesis of posttraumatic stress disorder. *Australian and New Zealand Journal of Psychiatry, 36*, 1–22.

Schore, A. (2002b). Advances in neuropsychoanalysis, attachment theory, and trauma research: Implications for self psychology. *Psychoanalytic Inquiry, 22*, 433–485.

Segalla, R. A. (1996). The unbearable embeddedness of being: Self-psychology, intersubjectivity and large group experience. *Group, 20*, 257–270.

Stern, D. (1985). *The interpersonal world of the infant: A view for psychoanalysis and developmental psychology*. New York: Basic Books.

Stern, D. P. (2001). Comments on the clinical material presented by Jill Scharff. *Psychoanalytic Inquiry, 21*, 499–507.

Stolorow, R. D. (2001). What in the (experiential) world is an "internal couple"? *Psychoanalytic Inquiry, 21*, 530–536.

Stolorow, R. D., & Atwood, G. E. (2002). *Contexts of being: The intersubjective foundations of psychological life*. Hillsdale, NJ: Analytic Press.

Stolorow, R. D., & Lachman, F. M. (1980). *Psychoanalysis of developmental arrests: Theory and treatment*. New York: International Universities Press.

Stone, W. N., & Gustafson, J. P. (1982). Technique and group psychotherapy of narcissistic and borderline patients. *International Journal of Group Psychotherapy, 32*, 29–42.

Szymborska, W. (1998). *Poems, new and collected, 1957-1997. Conversation with a stone* (pp. 62–64). New York: Harcourt Brace.

Wright, F. (1998). Discussion of "Difficult Patients." *International Journal of Group Psychotherapy, 48*, 339–345.

Yalom, I. D., & Yalom, M. (2021). *A matter of death and life*. Stanford, CA: Stanford University Press.

Index